Kathleen Swenson Miller, PhD, OTR/L
Georgiana L. Herzberg, PhD, OTR/L
Sharon A. Ray, ScD, OTR/L
Editors

Homelessness in America: Perspectives, Characterizations, and Considerations for Occupational Therapy

Homelessness in America: Perspectives, Characterizations, and Considerations for Occupational Therapy has been co-published simultaneously as *Occupational Therapy in Health Care,* Volume 20, Numbers 3/4 2006.

Pre-publication REVIEWS, COMMENTARIES, EVALUATIONS . . .

"A comprehensive examination of homelessness from an occupational therapy point of view . . . Chapters naturally flow from an overview of homelessness to an understanding of the phenomenon of homelessness, and then to occupational therapy application. . . . REQUIRED READING FOR ANY OCCUPATIONAL THERAPY PRACTITIONER WORKING WITH A HOMELESS POPULATION."

Victoria P. Schindler, PhD, OTR, FAOTA
Program Director and Associate Professor of Occupational Therapy
Richard Stockton College of New Jersey

More pre-publication
REVIEWS, COMMENTARIES, EVALUATIONS . . .

"Promises to stimulate new perspectives and programmatic ideas for therapists in the field, as well as a valuable introduction for those entering the field. Experts focus on occupational therapy philosophy, theory and practice as it relates to policy and service delivery for persons who are homeless. Practitioners will find a host of FRESH IDEAS for working with families, youths, and adults with mental illness, provided by knowledgeable occupational therapists who have extensive experience in their respective specialties. Content includes the occupational concerns of those who are homeless; use of the theory of Occupational Adaptation to understand the experience of people living in a homeless shelter; mother-toddler interactions in transitional housing; the role of occupational therapy in work with homeless youth; the use of the Model of Human Occupation with mothers in a homeless shelter; and life skills training for adults with mental illness who are homeless. Readers are exposed to a wide range of stimulating philosophical perspectives, as well as innovative yet practical programs. A MUST READ FOR ANYONE WHO WORKS WITH PERSONS WHO ARE HOMELESS."

Diana M. Bailey, EdD, OTR, FAOTA
Associate Professor
Tufts University

"As an experienced OT mental health practitioner and administrator working with homeless adults, I found the book **Homelessness in America** THOUGHT-PROVOKING AND HELPFUL to my practice. It approaches the complex issues of homelessness from multiple perspectives, ranging from theoretical concepts to pragmatic application. The chapters in the overview section offer clear explanations of how homelessness is viewed and how homeless services are delivered in our society. THIS IS ESSENTIAL INFORMATION FOR ANY PRACTITIONER who is interested in starting programs or initiating OT services with existing providers of homeless services. The book addresses also practice issues that are germane to targeted populations who represent a large and/or growing number of homeless individuals, single mothers with children, youth and mentally ill adults. Of particular interest to me were the chapters that describe the Canadian Occupational Performance Measure, an OT assessment tool that captures the unique cultural and functional challenges of homeless adults and can lead to meaningful goal setting. THE BOOK INFORMS AND INSPIRES US as OT practitioners to move forward to serve this underserved and often stigmatized population."

Peggy S. Sabol, MA, OTR/L
Manager, Psychiatry
(manager of 3 supportive housing programs)
Northwestern Memorial Hospital,
Ontario, Canada

Homelessness in America: Perspectives, Characterizations, and Considerations for Occupational Therapy

Homelessness in America: Perspectives, Characterizations, and Considerations for Occupational Therapy has been co-published simultaneously as *Occupational Therapy in Health Care*, Volume 20, Numbers 3/4 2006.

CENTRAL ARKANSAS LIBRARY SYSTEM
LITTLE ROCK PUBLIC LIBRARY
100 ROCK STREET
LITTLE ROCK, ARKANSAS 72201

Monographic Separates from *Occupational Therapy in Health Care*™

For additional information on these and other Haworth Press titles, including descriptions, tables of contents, reviews, and prices, use the QuickSearch catalog at http://www.HaworthPress.com.

Homelessness in America: Perspectives, Characterizations, and Considerations for Occupational Therapy, edited by Kathleen Swenson Miller, PhD, OTR/L, Georgiana L. Herzberg, PhD, OTR/L, and Sharon A. Ray, ScD, OTR/L (Vol. 20, No. 3/4, 2006). *"A comprehensive examination of homelessness from an occupational therapy point of view . . . Chapters naturally flow from an overview of homelessness to an understanding of the phenomenon of homelessness, and then to occupational therapy application. . . . REQUIRED READING FOR ANY OCCUPATIONAL THERAPY PRACTITIONER WORKING WITH A HOMELESS POPULATION." (Victoria P. Schindler, PhD, OTR, FAOTA, Program Director and Associate Professor of Occupational Therapy, Richard Stockton College of New Jersey)*

The Scholarship of Practice: Academic-Practice Collaborations for Promoting Occupational Therapy, edited by Patricia Crist, PhD, OTR/L, FAOTA, and Gary Kielhofner, DrPH, OTR, FAOTA (Vol. 19, No. 1/2, 2005). *"An excellent resource for any program pursuing collaborative, creative, and emerging practice opportunities. . . . Provides specific methods for a wide variety of applications. A must-read text!" (Kerry Muehler, MS, OTR/L, Assistant Professor and Academic Fieldwork Coordinator, Department of Occupational Therapy, University of South Dakota)*

Best Practices in Occupational Therapy Education, edited by Patricia A. Crist, PhD, OTR/L, FAOTA, and Marjorie E. Scaffa, PhD, OTR, FAOTA (Vol. 18, No. 1/2, 2004). *" A Valuable Resource for Educators. . . Provides practical examples of student learning experiences such as problem-based learning, the use of portfolios, brain teasers and online programs." (Kathleen Matuska, MPH, OTR/L, Associate Professor of Occupational Science and Occupational Therapy, College of St. Catherine, St. Paul, Minnesota)*

Occupational Therapy Practice and Research with Persons with Multiple Sclerosis, edited by Marcia Finlayson, PhD, OT(C), OTR/L (Vol. 17, No. 3/4, 2003). *Explores the complex OT issues arising from multiple sclerosis and suggests ways to enhance OT practice or research with people with MS.*

Interprofessional Collaboration in Occupational Therapy, edited by Stanley Paul, PhD, and Cindee Q. Peterson, PhD, OTR (Vol. 15, No. 3/4, 2001). *"A Good Source of Information. . . . Introduces the reader to the concept of interprofessional collaboration, its benefits, barriers, and strategies for developing such collaboration. . . . Presents a series of research studies that show the value of interprofessional collaboration to achieve outcomes at different levels and within different service delivery models." (Dyhalma Irizarry, PhD, OTR/L, FAOTA, Director, Occupational Therapy Program, University of Puerto Rico)*

Education for Occupational Therapy in Health Care: Strategies for the New Millennium, edited by Patricia Grist, PhD, OTR/L, FAOTA, and Marjorie Scaffa, PhD, OTR/L, FAOTA (Vol. 15, No. 1/2, 2001). *"Provides Truly Imaginative Ideas for preparing the practitioners of the near future–and not a moment too soon! It is easy to see that these authors have been outstanding clinicians. . . . they put their OT skills to work in creating these unique learning-by-doing educational packages. Especially exciting are the clever ways in which alternative sites and programs are used to provide fieldwork experiences." (Nedra P. Gillette, MEd, OTR, ScD (Hon), Director, Institute for the Study of Occupation and Health, American Occupational Therapy Foundation)*

Community Occupational Therapy Education and Practice, edited by Beth P. Velde, PhD, OTR/L, and Peggy Prince Wittman, EdD, OTR/L, FAOTA (Vol. 13, No. 3/4, 2001). *"Introduces the concept of community-based practice in non-traditional settings. Whether one is concerned with wellness and the aging process or with debilitating situations, injuries, or diseases such as homelessness, AIDS, or multiple sclerosis, this collection details the process of moving forward." (Scott D. McPhee, DrPH, OT, FAOTA, Associate Dean and Chair, School of Occupational Therapy, Belmont University, Nashville, Tennessee)*

CENTRAL ARKANSAS LIBRARY SYSTEM
LITTLE ROCK PUBLIC LIBRARY
100 ROCK STREET
LITTLE ROCK, ARKANSAS 72201

Homelessness in America: Perspectives, Characterizations, and Considerations for Occupational Therapy

Kathleen Swenson Miller, PhD, OTR/L
Georgiana L. Herzberg, PhD, OTR/L
Sharon A. Ray, ScD, OTR/L
Editors

Homelessness in America: Perspectives, Characterizations, and Considerations for Occupational Therapy has been co-published simultaneously as *Occupational Therapy in Health Care*, Volume 20, Numbers 3/4 2006.

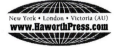

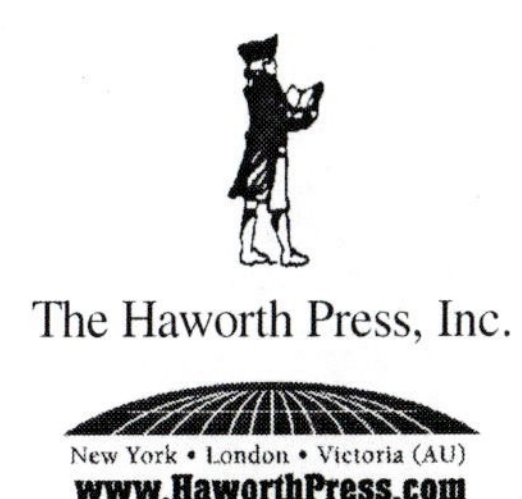

Homelessness in America: Perspectives, Characterizations, and Considerations for Occupational Therapy has been co-published simultaneously as *Occupational Therapy in Health Care*™, Volume 20, Numbers 3/4 2006.

© 2006 by The Haworth Press, Inc. All rights reserved. No part of this work may be reproduced or utilized in any form or by any means, electronic or mechanical, including photocopying, microfilm and recording, or by any information storage and retrieval system, without permission in writing from the publisher. Printed in the United States of America.

The development, preparation, and publication of this work has been undertaken with great care. However, the publisher, employees, editors, and agents of The Haworth Press and all imprints of The Haworth Press, Inc., including The Haworth Medical Press® and Pharmaceutical Products Press®, are not responsible for any errors contained herein or for consequences that may ensue from use of materials or information contained in this work. With regard to case studies, identities and circumstances of individuals discussed herein have been changed to protect confidentiality. Any resemblance to actual persons, living or dead, is entirely coincidental.

The Haworth Press is committed to the dissemination of ideas and information according to the highest standards of intellectual freedom and the free exchange of ideas. Statements made and opinions expressed in this publication do not necessarily reflect the views of the Publisher, Directors, management, or staff of The Haworth Press, Inc., or an endorsement by them.

Library of Congress Cataloging-in-Publication Data

Homelessness in America: perspectives, characterizations, and considerations for occupational therapy / Kathleen Swenson Miller, Georgiana L. Herzberg, Sharon A. Ray, editors.

p. ; cm.

"Co-published simultaneously as Occupational therapy in health care, v. 20, no. 3/4, 2006."

Includes bibliographical references and index.

ISBN-13: 978-0-7890-3191-4 (hard cover : alk. paper)

ISBN-10: 0-7890-3191-4 (hard cover : alk. paper)

ISBN-13: 978-0-7890-3192-1 (soft cover : alk. paper)

ISBN-10: 0-7890-3192-2 (soft cover : alk. paper)

1. Occupational therapy. 2. Mentally ill homeless persons. 3. Homelessness–United States. I. Swenson Miller, Kathleen. II. Herzberg, Georgiana L. III. Ray, Sharon A.

[DNLM: 1. Occupational Therapy–methods. 2. Homeless Persons.

W1 OC601H v.20 no.3/4 2006 / WB 555 H765 2006]

RC487.H66 2006

362.2086'942–dc22

2006025363

Indexing, Abstracting & Website/Internet Coverage

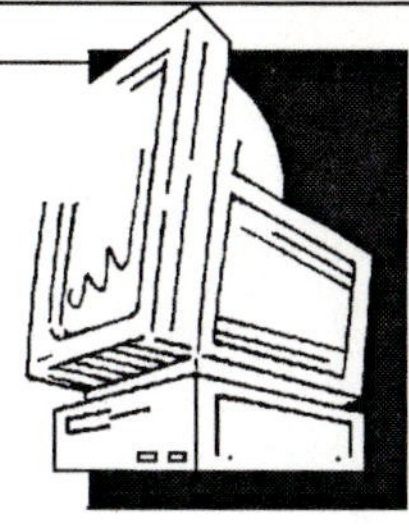

This section provides you with a list of major indexing & abstracting services and other tools for bibliographic access. That is to say, each service began covering this periodical during the year noted in the right column. Most Websites which are listed below have indicated that they will either post, disseminate, compile, archive, cite or alert their own Website users with research-based content from this work. (This list is as current as the copyright date of this publication.)

Abstracting, Website/Indexing Coverage . . . . Year When Coverage Began

- ***Abstracts in Social Gerontology: Current Literature on Aging (Sage)*** **1989**
- ***Biology Digest (in print & online) <http://www.infotoday.com>*** . **1990**
- ***Brandon/Hill Selected List of Journals in Allied Health Sciences <http://www.mssm.edu/library/brandon-hill >*** **2000**
- ***British Library Inside (The British Library) <http://www.bl.uk/services/current/inside.html>*** **2006**
- ***CINAHL (Cumulative Index to Nursing & Allied Health Literature) (EBSCO) <http://www.cinahl.com>*** **1987**
- ***CINAHL Plus (EBSCO)*** **2006**
- ***EBSCOhost Electronic Journals Service (EJS) <http://ejournals.ebsco.com>*** **2001**
- ***Elsevier EFlow-I*** **2006**
- ***Elsevier Scopus <http://www.info.scopus.com>*** **2005**
- ***EMBASE.com (The Power of EMBASE + MEDLINE Combined) <http://www.embase.com>*** **1984**

(continued)

- *EMBASE/Excerpta Medica Secondary Publishing Division. Included in newsletters, review journals, major reference works, magazines & abstract journals <http://www.elsevier.nl>* 1984
- *EMCare (Elsevier) <http://www.elsevier.com>* 2006
- *Exceptional Child Education Resources (ECER), (CD/ROM from SilverPlatter and hard copy) <http://www.ericec.org/ecer-db.html>* 1985
- *Google <http://www.google.com>*. 2004
- *Google Scholar <http://scholar.google.com>* 2004
- *Haworth Document Delivery Center <http://www.HaworthPress.com/journals/dds.asp>* 1984
- *Health & Psychosocial Instruments (HaPI) Database (available online and as a CD-ROM from Ovid Technologies)*. 1986
- *Index Copernicus <http://www.indexcopernicus.com>*. 2006
- *Human Resources Abstracts (Sage)* 1989
- *Index Guide to College Journals (core list compiled by integrating 48 indexes frequently used to support undergraduate programs in small to medium-sized libraries)* 1999
- *Links@Ovid (via CrossRef targeted DOI links) <http://www.ovid.com>*. 2005
- *MANTIS (Manual, Alternative & Natural Therapy). MANTIS is available through three database vendors: Ovid, Dialog & DataStar. In addition, it is available for searching through <http://www.healthindex.com>* 1999
- *Occupational Therapy Database (OTDBASE) has a user friendly index created so that each abstract can be found easily & quickly. Subscriptions can be obtained at <http://www.otdbase.org>* 1984
- *Occupational Therapy Index/AMED Database* 1993
- *OCLC ArticleFirst <http://www.oclc.org/services/databases/>* 2002
- *OCLC ContentsFirst <http://www.oclc.org/services/databases/>* . . 2002
- *OT SEARCH (American Occupational Therapy Foundation) <http://www.aota.org/otsearch/>* 1991
- *OTseeker <http://www.otseeker.com>* 2002

(continued)

- ***Ovid Linksolver (OpenURL link resolver via CrossRef targeted DOI links) <http://www.linksolver.com>*** **2005**
- ***Physiotherapy Evidence Database (PEDro) . . . . internet-based database of articles describing: a) randomized controlled trials; b) systematic reviews; c) evidence-based clinical practice guidelines, in physiotherapy related areas <http://www.pedro.fhs.usyd.edu.au>*** **2001**
- ***Scopus (see instead Elsevier Scopus) <http://www.info.scopus.com>*** **2005**
- ***Social Work Abstracts (NASW) <http://www.silverplatter.com/catalog/swab.htm>*** **1990**
- ***Ulrich's Periodicals Directory: International Periodicals Information Since 1932 (Bibliographic Access) <http://www.Bowkerlink.com>*** **2006**
- ***SwetsWise <http://www.swets.com>*** **2001**
- ***Violence and Abuse Abstracts (Sage)*** **1995**
- ***zetoc (The British Library) <http://www.bl.uk>*** **2004**

Special Bibliographic Notes related to special journal issues (separates) and indexing/abstracting:

- indexing/abstracting services in this list will also cover material in any "separate" that is co-published simultaneously with Haworth's special thematic journal issue or DocuSerial. Indexing/abstracting usually covers material at the article/chapter level.
- monographic co-editions are intended for either non-subscribers or libraries which intend to purchase a second copy for their circulating collections.
- monographic co-editions are reported to all jobbers/wholesalers/approval plans. The source journal is listed as the "series" to assist the prevention of duplicate purchasing in the same manner utilized for books-in-series.
- to facilitate user/access services all indexing/abstracting services are encouraged to utilize the co-indexing entry note indicated at the bottom of the first page of each article/chapter/contribution.
- this is intended to assist a library user of any reference tool (whether print, electronic, online, or CD-ROM) to locate the monographic version if the library has purchased this version but not a subscription to the source journal.
- individual articles/chapters in any Haworth publication are also available through the Haworth Document Delivery Service (HDDS).

ALL HAWORTH BOOKS AND JOURNALS
ARE PRINTED ON CERTIFIED
ACID-FREE PAPER

Homelessness in America: Perspectives, Characterizations, and Considerations for Occupational Therapy

CONTENTS

ABOUT THE EDITORS

Kathleen Swenson Miller, PhD, OTR/L, holds a baccalaureate degree in occupational therapy from the University of Minnesota, a master's degree in occupational therapy from Boston University, and a PhD in public health from Temple University in Philadelphia. She currently is a faculty member at Thomas Jefferson University, leads a graduate concentration in Community Health and Participation, and is a Research Associate in the Center for Collaborative Research at Thomas Jefferson University. Building upon her extensive experience in creating community programs, in maternal and child health, adolescent mental health, and understanding the impact of disability on occupational performance, Dr. Swenson Miller embarked on work with the homeless population nine years ago. She was the project director for several services grants working with the homeless population, served as a Program Evaluator for two transitional housing programs, and was a Project Director for two federal grants related to homelessness issues. She has presented nationally and published on models of community health, use of eHealth promotion with the homeless population, and work readiness with the homeless population. Her dissertation research focused on the social resources of the homeless population at two different points in the continuum of care. She has taken joy in introducing students to homeless persons who are working towards rebuilding their lives, erasing societal stereotypes of "who are the homeless."

Georgiana L. Herzberg, PhD, OTR/L, holds a baccalaureate degree in occupational therapy from Washington University in St. Louis (St. Louis, MO), a master's degree in vocational rehabilitation from Wayne State University (Detroit, MI), and a doctoral degree in higher adult and professional education from the University of Michigan (Ann Arbor, MI). She retired in 2005 as Professor of Occupational Therapy at Nova Southeastern University, Ft. Lauderdale, FL, where she taught about mental health practice and community issues in the master's and doctoral programs. Over the years, Dr. Herzberg published numerous articles on the issues of homelessness and presented both her research and program activities at local and national occupational therapy conferences, at national educational research conferences, and at two World Federation of Occupational Therapy conferences. She directed a four-year grant from the US Department of Health and Human Services, Health Resources and Services Administration (HRSA) from 2000-4 that created an interdisciplinary student training experience at a local shelter. She served on the Board of Directors of the Broward County Coalition to End Homelessness, Ft. Lauderdale, FL, from 1999-2005. She now lives in Jacksonville, FL.

Sharon A. Ray, ScD, OTR/L, received her BS degree in occupational therapy from the University of Pennsylvania. She received her MS degree and ScD degree from Boston University with a specialty in pediatrics. She has experience working with children and their families who have experienced homelessness through early intervention and school-based programs. She currently teaches pediatrics and electives on school-based practice at Tufts University, Boston School of Occupational Therapy. She provides consultation to pediatric occupational therapists, families, and to programs that provide therapeutic services to children with special needs. Her research involves examining parent-child interactions of families experiencing homelessness with a focus on the relationship to the child's engagement in activity.

She is a co-author of the *Guidelines for Provision of Occupational Therapy in Massachusetts Public Schools*. She also is a member of the administrative board for the Boston Institute for the Development of Infants and Parents (BIDIP).

OVERVIEW

The Status of Occupational Therapy: Addressing the Needs of People Experiencing Homelessness

Georgiana L. Herzberg, PhD, OTR/L
Sharon A. Ray, ScD, OTR/L
Kathleen Swenson Miller, PhD, OTR/L

SUMMARY. This paper discusses the move of occupational therapy practitioners towards providing services for people who are homeless, presents the results of an internet-based survey of assessment tools used with this population, and provides an overview of this volume's papers

Georgiana L. Herzberg is Retired, Professor of Occupational Therapy, Nova Southeastern University, Ft. Lauderdale, FL. Sharon A. Ray is Assistant Professor, Department of Occupational Therapy, Tufts University, Medford, MA. Kathleen Swenson Miller is Assistant Professor, Department of Occupational Therapy, Jefferson College of Health Professions, Thomas Jefferson University, Philadelphia, PA.

Address correspondence to: Georgiana Herzberg (E-mail: gherzberg@bellsouth.net).

[Haworth co-indexing entry note]: "The Status of Occupational Therapy: Addressing the Needs of People Experiencing Homelessness." Herzberg, Georgiana L., Sharon A. Ray, and Kathleen Swenson Miller. Co-published simultaneously in *Occupational Therapy in Health Care* (The Haworth Press, Inc.) Vol. 20, No. 3/4, 2006, pp. 1-8; and: *Homelessness in America: Perspectives, Characterizations, and Considerations for Occupational Therapy* (ed: Kathleen Swenson Miller, Georgiana L. Herzberg, and Sharon A. Ray) The Haworth Press, Inc., 2006, pp. 1-8. Single or multiple copies of this article are available for a fee from The Haworth Document Delivery Service [1-800-HAWORTH, 9:00 a.m. - 5:00 p.m. (EST). E-mail address: docdelivery@haworthpress.com].

Available online at http://othc.haworthpress.com
© 2006 by The Haworth Press, Inc. All rights reserved.
doi:10.1300/J003v20n03_01

while discussing the current status of occupational therapy interventions. doi:10.1300/J003v20n03_01 *[Article copies available for a fee from The Haworth Document Delivery Service: 1-800-HAWORTH. E-mail address: <docdelivery@haworthpress.com> Website: <http://www.HaworthPress.com>* *©2006 by The Haworth Press, Inc. All rights reserved.]*

KEYWORDS. Assessment, intervention, homeless

The purpose of this publication is to codify the current thinking of occupational therapy practitioners about interventions with people who are homeless and stimulate discussion about future directions. Homelessness is not unusual as an episodic, transitional, or chronic event in many of our clients' lives. People who are homeless experience health problems at more than twice the rate of persons in stable housing (Gelberg & Arangua, 2001). Forty-two percent of this population report activity limitations and 46% have chronic health conditions such as arthritis, diabetes, high blood pressure, or cancer (National Rehabilitation Hospital Center for Health & Disability Research, 2002; Burt, 2001). Women who are homeless experience poorer physical health than women in the general population and nearly 88% have a history of severe physical violence and/or sexual assault (Bassuk, Weinreb, Buckner, Browne, Salomon, & Bassuk, 1996). Families are now the fastest growing segment of this population and account for 41% of homeless people (U. S. Conference of Mayors, 2005). Their children have very high rates of acute illness, and are at increased risk for developmental delays, learning disabilities, emotional problems, cognitive impairments and behavioral problems (Better Homes Fund, 1999). People with severe and persistent mental illnesses are often caught in a spiral of downward economics that may include episodic, transitional, or chronic homelessness. Supplemental Security Income (SSI) is no longer a help in keeping people with mental or physical disabilities from becoming homeless because, in 2002, the average national rent exceeded the amount of income available for recipients of this federal program (Consortium for Citizens with Disabilities Housing Task Force, 2003). Persons with chronic health conditions and disabilities comprise populations with whom occupational therapy practitioners traditionally work so it becomes logical to also provide services in shelters and agencies that serve people who are homeless.

ASSESSMENTS USED BY OCCUPATIONAL THERAPISTS IN HOMELESS SHELTERS

In early 2005, the co-editors of this body of work conducted a survey of the assessment tools occupational therapy practitioners use with persons who are homeless. Via the Internet, print media, and personal contacts, we recruited a volunteer sample of practitioners working with people who are homeless. Requests for information appeared on three AOTA listservs (Community, Mental Health, and Program Director), in a private listserv (OT and Underserved Populations at YahooGroups.com), and in the on-line and print versions of OT Advance. No pediatric listservs were specifically contacted. Respondents provided contact information, credential (i.e., OT, OTA, other), current professional role, and indication if they worked with homeless adults, children, and/or families. Respondents then completed a survey of open-ended and forced choice questions to systematically provide information regarding (1) the use of both standardized tools and non-standardized/therapist-developed assessment tools, (2) the purpose for which each tool was used, (3) level of satisfaction with each identified tool, and (4) in the case of therapist-developed tools, if the person would be willing to share his/her assessment tool.

A total of 43 respondents (41 OT, 2 OTA) from 19 states in the US (AL, CA, CT, FL, IN, KY, LA, MI, MN, MT, NE, NM, NY, SD, TN, TX, VA, WA, and WI) and four countries (Canada, England, India, and Ireland) identified with an e-mail address. An additional four people (OT) provided no e-mail address and appeared to work with two of the respondents identified by e-mail addresses. Some respondents reported overlapping roles resulting in a role-defined total (n = 52) of four researchers, 32 clinicians, nine faculty members with academic responsibilities, two fieldwork coordinators, and five OT students. This group of people identified working in a total (n = 50) of 39 programs for adults, two programs for youth, four programs for children, and five programs for families. The limited responses related to work with children and families may reflect our recruitment method. For the adult population, there were 32 reports of the use of standardized assessments and 27 reports of the use of therapist-developed/non-standardized tools. See Table 1 for the most frequently used standardized assessments with adults and the purposes for which they are used.

Table 2 identifies single program use of standardized tools and Table 3 identifies the emphasis of therapist-developed, non-standardized tools in current use.

TABLE 1. Adult Program Most Frequently Used Standardized Assessment Tools and Their Purposes

Assessment Tool (frequency)	Purpose
KELS (16)	Daily living, self care, home management Community safety & money management Client needs for skills in independent living
ACL (12)	Cognitive ability related to work, ADLs, IADLs, Interpersonal communication Cognitive level of functioning Cognitive abilities and expectations of performance Problem solving abilities Level of supervision required How to teach clients with lower cognitive function
COPM (11)	Determining client goals Developing relevant client goals Client point of view about how functioning Client point of view about areas of dysfunction Determining client's view of important occupations Prioritizing interventions Building collaboration with client
OPHI-II (2)	Data to help plan life projects
Quality of Life Rating Scale (2)*	Important aspects of client's life and satisfaction

Note: n = 39 programs; All other standardized tools (n = 14 tools) were reported as used by only one program.
Allen Cognitive Levels (ACL), Canadian Occupational Performance Measure (COPM), Kohlman Evaluation of Living Skills (KELS), Occupational Performance History Interview-second version (OPHI-II)
Respondents were not specific regarding which of the many standardized quality of life rating scales (marketed for use with people with specific kinds of disabilities) were used.

The respondents who identified as working with the two youth programs reported use of the Adolescent Sensory Profile and an interest checklist. The assessment tools used in one or more of the four children's programs were the Sensory Profile, Developmental Test of Visual Motor Integration (VMI), and/or therapist-developed tools. The five programs for families reported using one or more of the following: Occupational Self-Assessment (OSA), Kohlman Evaluation of Living Skills (KELS),

TABLE 2. Standardized Assessment Tools Reported Used by a Single Program

Beck Depression Inventory
Occupational Self Assessment (OSA)
Nine Hole Peg Test
Adult Sensory Profile
Role Checklist
Functional Independence Measure (FIM)
Mini-Mental Status Examination (MMSE)
Rosenberg Self Esteem Scale
Barriers to Employment Success Scale
Occupational Circumstances Assessment Interview and Rating Scale (OCAIRS)
Bay Area Functional Performance Evaluation (BAFPE)
Ways of Coping
Contextual Memory Test

TABLE 3. Nonstandard or Therapist-Developed Tools Reported

ADL retraining (hygiene, safety, meal prep)
Center Developed questionnaires/Databases
Checklist of personal activities
Client interview
Client Self Assessment
Functional Assessment of Housing Needs
Functional Capacity Screen
Goal achievement scale adapted
Home safety assessment
Info taken from various tools (e.g., Board of Scientific Internet Tools)
Inventory of life skills
Living skills books (anger, stress, time management, money management, etc.)
OT Group Assessment
Screening of ADLs, domestic, & community skills
Screening of cognitive, vision, psychosocial performance, client goals, existing supports
Screening of self care, home management, upper extremity function
Self assessment of self care and productivity
Questionnaire related to Quality of Life Scale

Note: n = 27 responses from 21 programs

Canadian Occupational Performance Measure (COPM), Allen's Cognitive Levels (ACL), and/or therapist-developed tools.

Both the standardized and non-standardized tools reflect a clear concern for gathering information that allows collaborative development of client-centered interventions. The assessment tools also reflect a holistic concern for the contextual and performance factors that affect participation, allowing identification of strengths as well as challenges. The importance of client goals and priorities was readily apparent in the data and emphasized occupational performance and participation.

BEGINNING STAGES OF BUILDING A BODY OF LITERATURE

We have a sound beginning in documenting the work of occupational therapists with persons who are homeless, but the truth is that this is but a beginning. We are in the infant stages of creating a body of literature on how to collaborate with people who are homeless, to facilitate their occupational performance and their full participation in society. In these papers you will find that there is not a unified approach in assessment, in intervention, or in use of theory to help guide either assessment or intervention despite our clear emphasis on obtaining and using client input to guide interventions. These manuscripts do not reflect the age and gender majority demographics of homelessness. Our over-inclusion of articles reflecting interventions with children/youth and families (instead of adult males who represent 41% of the population who are homeless according to the US Conference of Mayors, 2005), reflects the government funding stream that allows occupational therapists to provide services for children. Such services can be reimbursed through the federal government's Head Start, early intervention, or school-based programs (IDEA, 2004). The over-inclusion also reflects, we believe, our profession's current emphasis on pediatric occupational therapy which accounts for 34% of all work environments of AOTA members (AOTA Workforce Trends Survey, 2003).

This body of work illuminates our current stage of trying to understand the phenomena of homelessness and occupational therapy roles. Hopefully, it will provide a baseline for dialog on our future directions, and stimulate healthy debate about–and interest in–an understanding of the occupational performance issues of persons who are homeless, occupational therapy practitioner roles, and evidence-based interventions that support full participation by this population. There is a substantial need for additional research focusing on outcomes measurement and on funder-defined outcomes measurement as is elaborated in the systems article by Livingston and Swenson-Miller in this publication.

This special volume provides an interface between occupational therapy philosophy, occupational therapy practice, research on issues of homelessness, and policy implications. In Articles 2 and 3, you will find discussion of the complex issues of homelessness and the systems of available services. In articles 4 through 8, the phenomenon of homelessness is explored using different occupational therapy theories and perspectives. Articles 9 through 12 include studies of occupational therapy assessments and interventions with persons who are homeless. You will read descriptions and research that increase understanding of how theoretical models, assessment instruments, and/or program evaluation techniques are used with persons who are homeless. These articles provide insights that can lead to societal inclusion, occupational participation, and social justice for this population.

We thank our guest editors for their thoughtful and insightful comments. Our guest editors are Laura Hansen, CEO of the Broward Coalition to End Homelessness, Ft. Lauderdale, FL; Kathleen Hagen, Educational Support Services, Nova Southeastern University, Ft. Lauderdale, FL; Debbie Perry, Director of Homeless Programs, Henderson Mental Health Services, Ft. Lauderdale, FL; Dr. Susan Kusama, retired occupational therapy educator, St. Louis, MO; Dr. Susan Toth-Cohen, Associate Professor, Department of Occupational Therapy, Thomas Jefferson University, Philadelphia, PA; and Dr. Kevin Lyons, Director of the Center for Collaborative Research, Thomas Jefferson University, Philadelphia, PA. We hope these articles will generate additional thinking about how participation is supported and generate new ideas on occupational therapy roles that facilitate health and wellness and ensure client-centered, culturally sensitive occupational therapy practice.

REFERENCES

Allen, C. K. (1997). *Allen Cognitive Level Screen*. Colchester, CT: S & S Worldwide.

American Occupational Therapy Association (2003). Workforce trends in Occupational Therapy. Available at http://www.aota.org/featured/area2/docs/4-1_Worktrends.pdf, Accessed 3/16/06.

Bassuk, E. L., Weinreb, L. F., Buckner, J. C., Browne, A., Salomon, A., & Bassuk, S. S. (1996). The characteristics and needs of sheltered homeless and low-income housed mothers. *Journal of the American Medical Association*, 276(8), 640-646.

Better Homes Fund. (1999). *America's homeless children: New outcasts.* Newton, MA: Author.

Burt, M. (2001). *Homeless families, singles, and others: Findings from the 1996 national survey of homeless assistance providers and clients.* Housing Policy Debate (Fannie Mae Foundation), 12, 737-780.

Consortium for Citizens with Disabilities Housing Task Force (2005). Priced Out in 2004: The housing crisis for people with disabilities. Available at http://www.c-c-d.org/pricedout04.pdf, Accessed 3/16/06.

Gelberg, L., Gallagher, T. C., Andersen, R. M. & Koegel, P. (1997). Competing priorities as a barrier to medical care among homeless adults in Los Angeles. *American Journal of Public Health 87*(2): 217-220.

Kielhofner, G., Mallison, T., Crawford, C., Nowak, M., Rigby, M., Henry, A., & Walens, D. (1997). *Occupational Performance History Interview–second version.* Bethesda, MD: AOTA Products.

Law, M., Baptiste, S., Carswell, A., McColl, M.A., Polatajko, H., & Pollock, N. (1998). *Canadian Occupational Performance Measure (3rd ed.).* Ottawa: CAOT Publications ACE.

McGourty, L. K. (1999). *Kohlman Evaluation of Living Skills.* Bethesda, MD: AOTA Products.

National Rehabilitation Hospital Center for Health & Disability Research (2002). Homeless and disabled: Focusing on the health and healthcare needs of an underserved population. Available at http://www.nrhrehab.org/documents/Research/brief_housing.pdf, Accessed 3/16/06.

U. S. Conference of Mayors (2005). A status report on hunger and homelessness in America's cities. Washington, DC: Author. Available at http://www.mayors.org/USCM/home.asp, Accessed 3/16/06.

doi:10.1300/J003v20n03_01

Homelessness: Perspectives, Misconceptions, and Considerations for Occupational Therapy

Terry Petrenchik, PhD, OTR/L, OT Reg. (Ont.)

SUMMARY. Like poverty, the problem of homelessness has been with us to varying degrees since the founding of our nation. Attempts to explain homelessness have an equally long history. Hence, the literature and popular media are home to divergent perspectives, explanations, and characterizations of homelessness. The objectives of this paper are to present a unifying taxonomy of prominent perspectives on homelessness, and to illustrate how various perspectives lead to particular characterizations of persons who become homeless. The taxonomy traces the connection between perspectives and interpretations of the problem and helps to illuminate implicit and often unexamined assumptions about who becomes homeless and why. Critical examination of these perspectives is vital because our individual and collective understanding of homelessness is a powerful determinant of how we approach occupational therapy practice with this population. Implications for community practice and program

---

Terry Petrenchik is Assistant Professor, School of Rehabilitation Science, McMaster University, 1400 Main St. West, Hamilton, Ontario, Canada L8S 1C7 (E-mail: petrent@mcmaster.ca).

[Haworth co-indexing entry note]: "Homelessness: Perspectives, Misconceptions, and Considerations for Occupational Therapy." Petrenchik, Terry. Co-published simultaneously in *Occupational Therapy in Health Care* (The Haworth Press, Inc.) Vol. 20, No. 3/4, 2006, pp. 9-30; and: *Homelessness in America: Perspectives, Characterizations, and Considerations for Occupational Therapy* (ed: Kathleen Swenson Miller, Georgiana L. Herzberg, and Sharon A. Ray) The Haworth Press, Inc., 2006, pp. 9-30. Single or multiple copies of this article are available for a fee from The Haworth Document Delivery Service [1-800-HAWORTH, 9:00 a.m. - 5:00 p.m. (EST). E-mail address: docdelivery@haworthpress.com].

Available online at http://othc.haworthpress.com
© 2006 by The Haworth Press, Inc. All rights reserved.
doi:10.1300/J003v20n03_02

planning for individuals and families in homeless shelters are also discussed. doi:10.1300/J003v20n03_02 *[Article copies available for a fee from The Haworth Document Delivery Service: 1-800-HAWORTH. E-mail address: <docdelivery@haworthpress.com> Website: <http://www.HaworthPress.com>* *©2006 by The Haworth Press, Inc. All rights reserved.]*

KEYWORDS. Homeless, occupational therapy, community practice

INTRODUCTION

Homelessness in America, unless precipitated by acts of terrorism or natural disasters, receives relatively little attention in the media. Consequently, like an iceberg floating at sea, the depth and breadth of the phenomenon of homelessness remains hidden from public view. The visible tip of homelessness, which resurfaced as a social concern in the 1980s (Burt, 1991), tends to elicit fervent rather than impartial reactions among citizens and scholars alike. For decades, centuries in fact, we as a nation and as citizens have debated the origins of homelessness in America.

Virtually everyone, from children to the elderly, and bus drivers to politicians, has an opinion on homelessness. Such a mixture of perspectives, which reflect our varied belief systems, values, and mores, can quickly heat and polarize social and scholarly discourses on homelessness. Genuinely impartial discussions about homelessness are rare, in part because this topic cuts to the very core of our personal and societal values.

Even knowledge derived from objective scientific research has an element of subjectivity. This is because disciplines, professions, and subgroups within them, are perspectivistic. That is, they see and interpret phenomena and human behavior from a shared orientation that is particular to that group. The collective identities, shared philosophies, and paradigms that unite disciplines and organize their scholarly work also encourage a shared and necessarily delimited view of social phenomena such as homelessness. Thus, the question of perspective should be a fundamental consideration in all attempts to understand and address the inherently value-laden issue of homelessness.

Occupational therapy is a relative newcomer to the matter of homelessness, particularly in the area of research. As consumers and, increasingly, as producers of research on homelessness, questioning the assumptions and perspectives underlying bodies of research is an essential practice. It is not enough to evaluate and grade the methodological rigor of research evidence. The willingness and ability to question the validity of collective assumptions and perspectives, our own and those of other disciplines, is vital. In science, we refer to perspectives as theories, models, or paradigms. As one wades through the literature on homelessness in pursuit of evidence and understanding, it is important to appreciate its historical milieu and to recognize the paradigms and methodologies popular in a given era. If not, we run the risk of perpetuating potentially outdated and perhaps harmful perspectives that may have little relevance in a rapidly changing world.

Critical examination rather than passive acceptance of prevalent perspectives on homelessness is vital because our individual and collective understanding of who becomes homeless and why is a powerful determinant of how we approach occupational therapy practice with this population. With this in mind, the objectives of this paper are to provide a taxonomy of prominent perspectives on homelessness, and to illustrate how various perspectives lead to particular characterizations of persons who become homeless. The paper concludes with a discussion of considerations for occupational therapy practice in homeless shelters.

HOMELESSNESS: CONTEXTUALIZING THE PROBLEM

This paper addresses everyday homelessness–the experience of being placeless and without a fixed residence for reasons other than a natural catastrophe or man-made disaster. Rarely, if ever, does this form of homelessness result from one or two discrete factors operating in isolation. Rather, everyday homelessness is an experience that arises from a confluence of factors including housing and labor market conditions, poverty, social and racial inequality, personal vulnerabilities, and precarious life circumstances (Baumohl, 1996; Burt, 2001).

Unlike other forms of homelessness, which are caused by extraordinary, transitory events within a particular geographic region (e.g., Hurricane Katrina), everyday homelessness is a ubiquitous and persistent dilemma. It is a nationwide problem, the size of which depends upon one's definition of homelessness and the methods used for estimating its prevalence (Burt, 1999). Using the federal definition of homelessness (See Livingston & Swenson Miller, this volume), and data from the 1996 National Survey of Homeless Assistance Providers and Clients (NSHAPC), Burt and colleagues (2001) estimate that as many as 3.5 million people, 1.4 million of whom are children, are likely to experience homelessness in a given year. Putting this figure into larger perspective, the estimated number of Americans who experience homelessness in any given year currently exceeds the combined annual incidence of new and recurrent cases of coronary attack and stroke (U.S. Centers for Disease Control and Prevention [CDC], 2005a, 2005b).

Although not everyone who experiences income poverty becomes homeless, the two problems are closely interrelated. Extreme poverty is a common thread that binds the otherwise diverse and shifting population of citizens who become homeless each year (Fosburg & Dennis, 1999). Poverty status dramatically increases the likelihood of experiencing at least one episode of homelessness (Burt, 2001). Once a person becomes homeless, income poverty and the social problems that coalesce in an environment of poverty increase the probability of experiencing repeat episodes of homelessness, particularly among female-headed single parent families (Burt). While income poverty alone does not explain the phenomenon of homelessness, subsistence level poverty is the defining context of homelessness. Therefore, a complete understanding of homelessness requires an appreciation of the antecedents and consequences of deep poverty.

TAXONOMY OF PERSPECTIVES ON HOMELESSNESS

Homelessness reemerged as a visible social concern in the early 1980s (Burt, 1991). During that time, two opposing explanations of homelessness were popular (Burt, Aron, Lee, & Valente, 2001). One view emphasized personal vulnerabilities as the principal cause of homelessness while the opposing view emphasized structural factors such as housing and labor markets. Today, there is general scholarly agreement that both personal and structural factors influence homelessness (Baumohl, 1996; Burt et al., 2001; Fosburg & Dennis, 1999). However, the pervasiveness and persistence of homelessness in America suggest that as a society we have yet to reach consensus on the root causes of homelessness.

Rank's (1994) taxonomy of welfare recipiency is a useful framework for organizing the divergent perspectives on homelessness found in the literature and in the media. These perspectives, which include structural, cultural, and intrapersonal views of homelessness (see Table 1) represent a broad continuum of ideas ranging from victim blaming to Marxism. Each of these perspectives reflects both the historical milieu and the prevailing behavioral and social sciences paradigm of the time. Thus, the purpose of the taxonomy appearing in Table 1 is to introduce chief aspects of structural, cultural and intrapersonal perspectives of homelessness.

TABLE 1. Structural, Cultural, and Intrapersonal Perspectives on Homelessness

Structural	Cultural	Intrapersonal
Dual Labor Market Theory – Posits two distinct labor markets operating under different rules, one of which leads to the subordination of women and vulnerable populations.	Culture of Poverty – Poverty leads to a self-perpetuating, intergenerational culture of alienation, present-time orientation, oppression, and dysfunction.	Attitudinal/Motivational – Lack of effort or thrift – Moral failing – Lack of talent or ability – Fecklessness – Promiscuity – Sense of entitlement
Functionalism – Institutions and social phenomena such as homelessness exist, because somehow they serve a function or a purpose in society.	Social Isolation – Social dislocation – Presence of social structural constraints and a lack of opportunity	Human Capital – Poor labor related skills and abilities – Lack of knowledge, education, and training
Big Brother Argument – Public assistance, welfare, and charity create work disincentives. – Government intrusions into private initiative must be curtailed in order to force individuals to work themselves out of poverty.		
Marxism – Systematic poverty and homelessness are inherent in the economic structure of capitalism.		

Note: Adapted from Rank, M. R. (1994). *Living on the edge: The realities of welfare in America.* New York: Columbia University Press.

Structural Perspective

From a structuralist perspective, everyday homelessness is primarily a product of structural factors. These include housing and labor markets, public policy, the removal of institutional supports for people with severe mental illness, the dismantling of social safety net programs, and racial, ethnic, and class discrimination (Baumohl, 1996; Burt, 2001; Fosburg & Dennis, 1999). In this view, homelessness is a condition created by a host of interrelated factors and circumstances that are external to individuals and families.

Housing and Labor Markets

Steep increases in housing prices and rent burdens, in combination with declining wages and a critical shortage of affordable housing, sets the stage for homelessness to occur (Burt et al., 2001; Koegel, Burnam, & Baumohl, 1996). Increasing rent burdens in combination with the growing disparity between the federal minimum wage and a living wage means housing at Fair Market Rents are out of reach for millions of Americans (National Low Income Housing Coalition [NLIHC], 2005). A living wage refers to the hourly wage necessary for a person to achieve a basic standard of living (e.g., housing, food, utilties, transportation, and basic medical care) while working 40 hours a week.

Working full time no longer guarantees escape from housing affordability problems, because wages have not kept pace with rising housing costs. Since 1997, the federal minimum wage has remained $5.15 per hour. The national housing wage for 2005, the wage needed to afford a two-bedroom rental unit at Fair Market Rent, is $15.78 per hour (NLIHC, 2005). This figure is more than three times the prevailing minimum wage. Though Fair Market Rents vary by geographic region, they are calculated according to the nationally accepted standard of paying no more than 30% of household income for housing costs. As in previous years, there is currently no location in the United States where a full-time minimum wage job provides enough income for a household to afford Fair Market Rent for a two-bedroom apartment (NLIHC).

A steep decline in the nation's stock of affordable housing also plays a significant role in creating the conditions for homelessness to occur. Between 1973 and 1993, the nation lost 2.2 million low-rental units (Bipartisan Millennial Housing Commission [MHC], 2002). In 2001, nearly 28 million households, or one in four households, spent more than 30% of their income on housing. One in seven households, or 14.4 million American families, had critical housing needs. That is, they paid more than half their household's income for housing and/or lived in substandard conditions (Lipman, 2002).

Social Policies

The current policy theme of tranferring power from the federal government to indivdual states to resolve social issues has translated into budget caps and cuts for several major social programs including federal aid for low-income housing, Medicaid, and child welfare. Federal policy changes, social program realignments, and budget cuts come at a difficult time for state governments struggling to balance their own budgets.

While aggregate state budget deficits have declined from $80 billion in fiscal year 2003-2004, to the current deficit of approximately $36 billion (McNichol, 2005), budget shortfalls continue to threaten state funded services. In recent years, states have resorted to spending cuts to social welfare programs for the poor, as well as reducing budgets for elementary, secondary and higher education (McNichol). Many low-income children who are homeless or precariously housed receive much needed school-related assistance (e.g., lunch, transportation, and special services) through the educational system by way of the McKinney-Vento Education for Homeless Children and Youth Program (1987).

Coalitions, researchers, and policy analysts concerned with the issues of poverty and homelessness cite the deterioration of social safety net programs and a lack of federal initiative as important structural factors contributing to the creation and perpetuation of homelessness. Low-income families with children who qualify for means-tested public assistance programs are especially hard hit by reductions in social welfare programs. Reduced assistance creates further hardship in low-income families already struggling to meet family needs for shelter, food, medical care, and other necessities. For these families, even small reductions in public assistance draw them one step closer to homelessness (Burt et al., 2001). Loss of public assistance among low-income families not only helps to create the condition of family homelessness, it also helps to prolong these episodes and predisposes families to recurrent episodes of homelessness (Fosburg & Dennis, 1999; Fremstad, 2004).

Cultural Perspective

Whereas the structural perspective situates the problem of homelessness in environmentally mediated circumstances beyond the control of individuals, the cultural perspective emphasizes familial and community culture as principal determinates of homelessness and poverty (Lewis, 1966; Moynihan, 1965). Cultural perspectives include the idea of a "culture of poverty," which stems from ethnographic studies by Lewis

(1966). In this view, circumstances such as poverty, homelessness, single motherhood, and welfare dependency represent a heritable "tangle of pathology" (Moynihan) transmitted via cultural norms. Moreover, this culture of poverty is purported to be self-perpetuating and intergenerational, thereby creating and sustaining a disadvantaged subculture.

From this perspective, homelessness and its associated problems originate from culturally transmitted deficiencies and engrained pathologies. In other words, homelessness is a product of the inherited traits of a self-perpetuating underclass (Handler, 1992). The culture of poverty argument, prevalent during the 1960s and early 1970s, is now widely regarded as a form of stereotyping and victim blaming (Handler; Huston, 1991; Luthar, 1999).

William J. Wilson (1996), a sociologist and leading scholar of urban poverty, posits a counter argument to the culture of poverty hypothesis. Wilson describes how various forms of economic and social disadvantage concentrate in jobless, low-income urban neighborhoods, resulting in a culture of disenfranchisement and social isolation. In his view, unflattering behaviors

> . . . often represent cultural adaptation to the systematic blockages of opportunities in the environment of the inner city and the society as a whole. These adaptations are reflected in habits, skills, styles, and attitudes shaped over time. (p. 72)

Wilson's analysis acknowledges an association between poverty and culture but avoids overtones of victim blaming and the extremism of the culture of poverty hypothesis. For Wilson, behaviors and cultures will change when structural conditions change. In this view, for homelessness to end, so must the social conditions that create joblessness, systematic poverty, and racial inequality.

Although we tend to shy away from these topics to avoid accusations of victim blaming and stereotyping, understanding the role of cultural and intrapersonal factors in homelessness and poverty has merit (Huston, 1991; Luthar, 1999). The key is designing balanced, thoughtful, and culturally sensitive investigations that include but do not lopsidedly focus on cultural influences and personal vulnerabilities. As both Huston and Luthar have suggested, understanding the effects of personal, cultural, and structural factors has important implications for program design and interventions aimed at alleviating poverty and homelessness.

Intrapersonal Perspective

The intrapersonal perspectives appearing in Table 1 fall into two categories: (a) attitudinal/motivational, and (b) human capital. To varying degrees, both of these perspectives reflect the notion that people who are homeless are somehow responsible for creating their own hardship. The stereotypical image of an apathetic welfare recipient who is unwilling to work is a familiar example of an attitudinal/motivational explanation of poverty and homelessness. Nowhere is this thinking more evident than in the entrenched and distorted notion that welfare recipiency is a preferred lifestyle among a majority of low-income single mothers. Although a comprehensive study of welfare recipiency (Rank, 1994) effectively debunked this myth, low-income mothers of minority status continue to encounter this stereotypical misrepresentation of their character and worth.

The myth that homelessness is fundamentally attributable to personal inadequacies and/or a lack of initiative is etched deeply in the American psyche. Stereotypical images of bag ladies, drunken vagrants, malingerers, beggars, and welfare mothers vivify the stigmatizing effects of characterizing homelessness as personal pathology. In the 1980s, researchers characterized homelessness as a mental health problem which inadvertently gave rise to a new stereotype–the caricature of homelessness as a psychotic single adult (Robertson & Greenblatt, 1992).

Attributing homelessness to personal inadequacies, moral failings, or a lack of initiative leads to judgments about whether and to what extent persons who are homeless deserve assistance. Historically, those we view as the deserving poor (e.g., the elderly, persons with disabilities, and children) are eligible for entitlements such as Social Security, Medicare/Medicaid, and disability benefits. Those we view as having created personal adversity due to vice, or the undeserving poor (Handler, 1992), oftentimes find themselves outside the eligibility criteria for various forms of public assistance and relief. This is especially true for single adult males (Burt et al., 2001).

From a personal pathology perspective, reformation of the individual, rehabilitation, and rectification of deviance are the primary mechanisms for eliminating or minimizing homelessness. On the policy front, welfare reform legislation known as the Personal Responsibility and Work Opportunity Reconciliation Act (1996) is an example of a federal initiative aimed at reformation of the individual. Although this legislation effectively ended unlimited public assistance, the reform system has failed to ensure that people moving off the welfare rolls are moving into stable, financially viable jobs with basic benefits. As a result, increased hardship and a greater risk of homelessness among low-income families have become unintended consequences of welfare reform (Fremstad, 2004).

Unquestionably, intrapersonal factors are relevant for understanding why, given similar circumstances, some adults and families become homeless while others do not. Ignoring the role of human capital and personal vulnerabilities would be naive because a lack of human capital–education, training, job skills, literacy and work experience, is evident in virtually every study of homelessness that collects such data. As well, mental illness, physical disabilities, substance abuse, and domestic violence are commonplace in this population (Burt et al., 2001; Fosburg & Dennis, 1999). However, human capital and personal vulnerabilities alone do not explain widespread homelessness in America (Burt, 2001). Emergent perspectives suggest the most reasonable explanation of homelessness lies between the two extremes of structuralism and personal vulnerabilities.

Structural Vulnerability: An Emergent Perspective

Among scholars of homelessness and its causes, the person versus environment debate is no longer tenable. Generally, there is acceptance that homelessness results from a complex interplay of personal vulnerabilities and structural factors (Baumohl, 1996; Burt et al., 2001; Fosburg & Dennis, 1999; Rog, 2002). Applying Rank's (1994) taxonomy, this perspective constitutes a structural vulnerability explanation of homelessness. From a structural vulnerability perspective, personal vulnerabilities matter to the extent they predict who is most at risk for becoming homeless. Structural factors matter to the extent they increase the likelihood that homelessness will occur. From this ecological, person-in-environment perspective the fundamental questions become (a) which particular person-environment configurations predict homelessness among vulnerable groups of individuals and families, and (b) which configurations are most important for ensuring residential stability?

In addressing these questions, Burt and colleagues (2001) have found that particular combinations of structural and personal factors influence the risk and geographical distribution of homelessness. In general, Burt (2001) concluded, "once structural factors have created the conditions for homelessness, personal factors can increase a person's vulnerability to losing his or her home . . . [but] without the presence of structural fault lines, personal vulnerabilities could not produce today's high levels of homelessness" (p. 2).

Which structural and personal factors figure prominently into this equation? Structural factors include a lack of affordable housing, declining wages, reductions in social safety net programs (e.g., welfare reform and removal of institutional supports for people with severe mental illness), a shrinking labor market for people with less than a college (or high school) education, and racial inequality and discrimination. On the other side of the equation are personal factors such as limited education or skills training, mental or physical disabilities, a lack of social support or social networks, substance abuse, and poverty (Burt, 2001; Rog, 2002). However, the combination and relative significance of these factors tend to vary in relationship to the outcome of interest (e.g., chronic versus episodic homelessness), the demographic composition of the sample (e.g., single adults versus families) and geographic location (e.g., urban versus rural).

A structural vulnerability explanation of homelessness, although not articulated as such, has garnered support among researchers and policy analysts (Burt et al., 2001; Fosburg & Dennis, 1999). However, public policy and attitudes oftentimes lag behind current thinking in the health, behavioral and social sciences. Historically, and at present, public policies concerning homelessness are subject to prevailing political ideologies and to socially constructed notions of the "deserving" and "undeserving" poor (Baumohl, 1996; Handler, 1992).

In summary, perspectives are the filters or lens though which we view and delimit an issue. That is, a perspective sets the limits of what we are able to see and to recognize as a possible reality. Understanding the entirety of a matter such as homelessness requires a willingness to examine issues from a variety of perspectives because each contributes to our understanding of the whole. Applying Rank's (1994) taxonomy of welfare recipiency to the issue of homelessness is useful because it allows us to view the problem from multiple angles. It also helps to illuminate the connection between perspectives and interpretations of the problem by clarifying implicit and often unexamined assumptions about who becomes homeless and why.

CHARACTERIZATIONS OF HOMELESSNESS

One of the principal aims of scientific research is to articulate and test paradigms or mini-theories about particular phenomena (Chambers, 1999). The caveat that is all paradigms, no matter how elegant, contain some level of inconsistency and incongruity because at best paradigms *approximate* reality.

While shared, unifying paradigms are essential for guiding scientific activity, they inevitably encourage a type of consensus reality that at times has unintentionally promoted a distorted view of persons who are homeless. Rosencheck and colleagues (1999) caution that use of descriptive classifications in research on homelessness (e.g., mentally ill, substance user, etc.), while necessary for identifying the specific needs of that particular subgroups, has the unintended consequence of reinforcing discrimination and stereotypical thinking about persons who become homeless. Snow, Anderson, and Koegel (1994) argue that a collective overreliance on psychopathology and disability perspectives, in combination with methodological shortcomings, has resulted in research that presents a distorted, decontextualized, and pathologized understanding of men, women, and children who experience homelessness.

Similarly, the evaluation tools used in research and professional practice have the power to redefine how people see themselves and how others see them. In other words, people are transformed "by assigning them to various categories (genius, slow learner, drug-free, etc.), where they are then treated, act, and come to think of themselves according to expectations associated with those categories" (Hanson, 1993, p. 294).

Conversely, research has played a valuable role in debunking myths and stereotypes about persons who become homeless. Public attitudes about women with children who become homeless are a case in point. Traditionally, these women have been portrayed as drug users, prostitutes, and welfare recipients who are less educated and more ill (physically and mentally) than their housed counterparts (Merves, 1992). The public view of mothers who end up on the streets or in a homeless shelter with their children is one of a bad parent who is incapable of providing her children with the love, care, and support they need. It is the image of personal failure resulting from one's own vices and inadequacies.

In contrast to stereotypes, research shows female-headed single parent families who become homeless are demographically similar to housed, income-poor families in terms of educational attainment, employment patterns, and maternal concern for child safety and well-being (Shinn & Weitzman, 1996). While parents in families who become homeless do report a greater frequency of substance abuse and mental health difficulties in comparison with parents in housed, income-poor families, these frequencies are well below rates reported by single adults who are homeless (Shinn & Weitzman). Additionally, families who experience homelessness tend to report greater income poverty and fewer housing subsidies in comparison with their housed counterparts (Shinn & Weitzman; U. S. Department of Health and Human Services [HHS], 1998).

While research has the potential to dispel public myths and stereotypes about homelessness, an overreliance on psychopathology and disability perspectives, and the language used to describe them, inadvertently helps to propagate the incomplete and pathologized portrait of homelessness found in the literature. The language used to communicate these perspectives is critical because language creates impressions and imparts meaning.

Language is a powerful social tool–it shapes how people think, act, and feel (Spaniol & Cattaneo, 1997). The words researchers and practitioners use to characterize and describe people and phenomena create powerful and lasting impressions of entire groups of human beings. We transmit these impressions to subsequent generations of researchers and practitioners through the literature we produce and through the professional stories that we share. In this way, lines of thinking and ways of knowing become reinforced and entrenched.

Traditionally, research involving individuals and families who are homeless, and the message it conveys, emphasizes disability and pathology. Consequently, summarizing the literature on homelessness for virtually any subgroup (e.g., single adults, families, or youth), inevitably results in a lopsided portrait of disability, psychopathology, and dysfunction. Countering this imbalance with research evidence is difficult because relatively little work has focused on the strengths and abilities of individuals and families who become homeless. This does not suggest we should abandon one extreme viewpoint in favor of another. Instead, adopting an ecological outlook, which emphasizes a balanced, contextualized representation of issues, would help to build a more complete body of literature on homelessness.

CONSIDERATIONS FOR OCCUPATIONAL THERAPY

Historically, occupational therapists have approached practice with a predominant focus on disease, injury, and impairment, and to a lesser extent, human environments. Although occupational therapists define environments broadly (American Occupational Therapy Association [AOTA], 2002; Canadian Association of Occupational Therapists [CAOT]), 1997; Law, 1991), in practice, there has been a strong tendency to focus primarily on aspects of the physical environment with relatively less attention given to the social, cultural, institutional, and economic environments that facilitate or constrain participation in everyday occupations. In effect, person-environment practice has lingered at the margins of direct practice, while performance component oriented interventions, which emphasize impairment and disability, have occupied center stage. In the 1990s, a slow but steady movement towards holistic, person-environment practice, which began in the 1970s, gained footing within the profession.

Recently, enabling participation became the stated objective of occupational therapy interventions in North America (AOTA, 2002; CAOT, 1997). By definition, to participate is to take part, to have a share of, or to share in with others (Merriam-Webster's Dictionary, 2003). Implicit in this definition is the notion of inclusion or membership in a larger whole. In a very real sense, inclusion, or where one stands in relationship to others and society, is a powerful determinant of the form, scope, and quality of one's participation in everyday occupations. Indeed, participation itself is not inherently beneficial, enjoyable, or meaningful. Rather, the configuration, quality, and suitability of the circumstances and environments in which individuals participate are instrumental in determining whether participation in everyday occupations contributes positively or negatively to a person's health and developmental outcomes.

Participation is an amalgam of occupation, environmental context, personal attributes, and subjective meaning. The fit among these interconnected elements, which change in dynamic relationship to one another, shapes the outcome of participation. In other words, participation is a product of on-going transactions between a person and his or her physical and social environments (Bronfenbrenner, 1979; Forsyth & Jarvis, 2002). Because the construct of participation is complex and multidimensional, fulfilling our role as enablers of participation will require both a deeper understanding of person-environment-occupation relations and an emphasis on enabling participation and occupational performance rather than on discrete skill-building.

Occupational therapy interventions with persons who are homeless typically occur in shelter environments (Griner, in press). The mandate of shelters, specifically transitional shelters, is to move residents into permanent housing within 24 months or less (McKinney-Vento Homeless Assistance Act, 1987). Thus, shelters can be service intensive settings in which resident participation in designated services is often compulsory and monitored (Barrow & Zimmer, 1999). Obligatory life skills training, social skills training, parenting classes, work readiness, and housing readiness programs are commonplace in homeless shelters. Because shelter programs tend to operate from a deficit model perspective, services in these environments tend to emphasize remediation of poor basic skills and rehabilitation (Barrow & Zimmer, 1999; Feins & Fosburg, 1999). With a culture of paternalism and reductionism so commonplace in homeless shelters, occupational therapists working in these settings must be vigilant about providing holistic, client-centered occupational therapy.

Ultimately, the goal of skills remediation programs in shelter environments is changes in performance and behavior through hierarchical skill development. Alternatively, or in combination, clients may receive instruction in health education and health promotion strategies. If they are parents, residents may also receive developmental health information about their child. The belief among skills remediation advocates is that skill gains through practice and instruction will ultimately translate into improvements in self-sufficiency and behavioral health outcomes. Yet, social sciences and behavioral health research clearly shows that interventions aimed principally at changing personal behaviors, habits, and lifestyles are often costly and ineffective (Smedley & Syme, 2000). Equally important, investigations have not found service-intensive, deficit model approaches to be effective for improving housing outcomes among persons exiting homelessness (Wong, Culhane, & Kuhn, 1997; Wong & Piliavin, 1997).

An alternative approach for occupational therapists is to focus on enabling participation by identifying and minimizing occupational performance barriers and environmental constraints, and by expanding opportunities for mastery experiences in a person's natural environment. In this approach, the emphasis is on maximizing goodness-of-fit among individuals, their occupations, and the socio-physical environments in which occupations occur. From this perspective, person-environment-occupation *relations* become the foci of research, assessment and intervention. This approach is in keeping with current thinking in the health sciences (Halfon & Hochstein, 2002; World Health Organization, 2001) and in the behavioral and social sciences (Smedley & Syme, 2000), all of which advocate an ecological or social environmental approach to health-related interventions.

Therapy models, which have been a mainstay of occupational therapy practice (Fidler, 2000), tend to have limited utility in community practice settings with marginalized and vulnerable populations (McKnight, 1995, 1997). Therapy models of practice, which are widely used in rehabilitation, focus on restoration of, or improvement in, the skills and abilities of an individual. In contrast, ecological practice frameworks emphasize person-environment-occupation fit, which discourages performance component oriented practice by focusing on the relationship among individuals, their occupations, and their environments. Like a structural vulnerability view of homelessness, ecological approaches balance the attention given to personal and environmental factors.

Ecological practice approaches do not ignore the important interrelationships among performance components, personal skills and abilities, and occupational performance. Rather, person-environment practice changes the way we approach and organize occupational therapy interventions. Therapy models rely on a bottom-up approach to achieve changes in occupational performance through hierarchical skill development. These approaches begin at the impairment level and work to restore and improve the skills and processes that underlie occupational performance (Weinstock-Zlotnick & Hinojosa, 2005). The belief is that skill gains will ultimately translate into improved occupational performance. Hence, the term bottom-up.

Conversely, top-down approaches begin at the level of occupational performance or participation. These interventions identify occupational performance barriers at the level of participation, in the natural environments where activities and occupations occur. The aim is to remove barriers to and expand opportunities for participation by first attending to affordances in the proximal environment. Environmental affordances are the real and perceived opportunities and actions allowed by the environment in specific relationship to an individual (Gibson, 1979; Norman, 1988). The second step involves progressively modifying the dynamic demands of an activity or occupation. Lastly, when necessary, a person's skills and abilities receive attention, but this is subsequent to addressing environmental affordances and the demands of the occupation. The emphasis here is on maximizing person-environment-occupation fit. In a top-down approach, discrete skill-building is the intervention of last choice.

Additionally, designing interventions to enable the participation of persons living in homeless shelters requires practitioners to shed an expert role within a medical model of practice and to adopt the role of collaborator, facilitator, and partner within a community-built model of practice. The distinction between community-based and community-built practice is an important one. Community-based practice simply relocates an expert model of practice into a community setting. Conversely, community-built practice attempts to equalize power relationships by using a participatory model to create effective and authentic partnerships (Labonte, 1997). In turn, authentic partnerships support client autonomy and choice, and build client capacities by assisting individuals to identify their own needs and assets, make choices, and develop strategies to make desired changes in their lives.

Community-built practice challenges occupational therapists to collaborate rather than to prescribe. The focus shifts from fixing problems and correcting deficits to enabling participation in everyday occupations by maximizing person-environment-occupation fit. Occupational therapists interested in community-built practice with persons who are homeless will be challenged to develop a deeper understanding of capacity-building approaches, environments, occupations, and the fundamentals of participation. This new role requires a shift from performance component oriented practice to an ecological model of practice, which focuses on the relationship, or fit among individuals, their occupations, and their environments.

The overarching goal of occupational therapy interventions for persons living in homeless shelters is to maximize person-environment-occupation fit to enable participation in the immediate shelter environment and to reconfigure person-environment-occupation relations to enable greater participation in the community. Occupational therapy interventions that give equal consideration to both personal and environmental factors are congruent with current thinking, concerning homelessness and health-related interventions, which emphasizes it is the *interplay* among factors, rather than the discrete factors themselves that merits our utmost attention. The challenge for occupational therapists will be to translate these theoretical concepts into informed, theory-driven person-environment interventions such as the one offered next.

Research has shown that a return to stable housing is a *prerequisite* to community participation for individuals and families experiencing homelessness (Rog & Holupka, 1999). In terms of program planning, this means attention to housing needs and related supports should come first, before addressing other issues. A return to housing is a critical first step in enabling community participation, or "getting back to the job market, getting hooked up with needed services, and reestablishing or initially establishing ties with family and other sources of support" (Rog & Holupka, p. 11:8). In short, research suggests that our principal aim as occupational therapists should be assisting individuals and families to return to housing and connecting them with the supports and services needed to improve residential stability and community participation over time. These findings challenge occupational therapists to take an active role in collaborating with service provider agencies to design and evaluate comprehensive housing-based programs and services.

Though the nation's homeless shelter system is a current necessity and serves as an important social safety net for the tens of thousands of citizens who become homeless each year, we should work to minimize the time individuals and families spend in shelter environments. While working in these settings, let us focus our efforts on creating environments and opportunities that foster resilience and human dignity in those among us who experience, firsthand, the harsh realities of deep poverty and social inequality.

CONCLUSION

Perspectives on homelessness and the language used to describe them matter a great deal. Beliefs and assumptions about the causes of homelessness shape both our societal response to this problem and our personal reactions when we encounter individuals who are homeless. Perspectives also sway our judgments about whether and to what extent persons who are homeless deserve assistance. Critical examination of our perspectives and their underlying assumptions is of fundamental importance because these orientations underpin our individual and collective response to the sociopolitical problem of homelessness in America.

Using Rank's (1994) taxonomy of welfare recipiency to organize divergent perspectives on homelessness into four prominent viewpoints is useful for several reasons. First, the varied perspectives captured in this taxonomy underscore the multifaceted nature of the enduring problem of homelessness. Second, the taxonomy makes it easier to see the linkages between perspectives and interpretations of a problem. Third, the taxonomy helps to clarify the assumptions that underlie various points of view about who becomes homeless and why. Understanding the viewpoints presented in the taxonomy (structural, cultural, intrapersonal, and structural vulnerability) are worthwhile because each leads to a particular characterization and understanding of persons who become homeless. How we comprehend the problem of homelessness shapes our beliefs about the viability and merit of possible solutions.

Acknowledgment of homelessness as a pressing social concern carries an associated responsibility to take corrective action. Thus, our immediate concern should be for the more than 800,000 men, women, and children who will be homeless tonight in America (Burt, 2001). A portion of these citizens will sleep in shelters while many others will sleep in cars, alleys, parks, or doubled up in the home of a friend or a relative. A large percentage of these individuals and families will be homeless for only a few weeks or months. Others will be homeless for years and many will experience recurrent episodes of homelessness.

Living homeless in America is a dangerous, debasing, and unhealthy experience that warrants national attention. Certainly, the best course of action is preventing homelessness before it occurs. Current realities (e.g., shortages of affordable housing, declining wages, reductions in social safety net programs, shrinking labor markets, and racial inequality) make it clear that a coherent national strategy is essential for preventing and ending homelessness.

Concerted action is also required at the local level because community-based strategies and agencies, both public and private, form the final safety net for the ranks of beleaguered citizens who become homeless each year. With appropriate training, occupational therapists can make a positive contribution at both the national and regional level, as well as in direct service to persons experiencing homelessness. The primary goal of occupational therapy programs and services for persons who are homeless, whether at the systems level or the individual level, is assisting fellow citizens to return to and participate in the economy, their community, and in society as a whole.

REFERENCES

American Occupational Therapy Association (2002). Occupational therapy practice framework: Domain and process. *American Journal of Occupational Therapy, 56*, 609-639.

Barrow, S., & Zimmer, R. (1999). Transitional housing and services: A synthesis. In L. Fosburg & D. Dennis (Eds.), *Practical lessons: The 1998 national symposium on homelessness research* (pp. 10:11-31). Washington, DC: U.S Department of Housing and Urban Development and U.S. Department of Health and Human Services.

Baumohl, J. (1996). *Homeless in America.* Phoenix, AZ: Oryx Press.

Bipartisan Millennial Housing Commission (2002). *Meeting our nation's housing challenges.* Washington, DC: Author.

Bronfenbrenner, U. (1979). *The ecology of human development: Experiments by nature and design.* Cambridge, MA: Harvard University Press.

Burt, M. R. (1991). Causes of the growth of homelessness during the 1980s. *Housing Policy Debate, 2*(3), 903-936.

Burt, M. R. (1999). Demographics and geography: Estimating needs. In L. Fosburg & D. Dennis (Eds.), *Practical lessons: The 1998 national symposium on homelessness research* (pp. 1:1- 24). Washington, DC: U. S. Department of Housing and Urban Development.

Burt, M. R. (2001). *What will it take to end homelessness?* Washington, DC: The Urban Institute.

Burt, M., Aron, L., Lee, E., & Valente, J. (2001). *Helping America's homeless: Emergency shelter or affordable housing?* Washington, DC: Urban Institute Press.

Canadian Association of Occupational Therapists (1997). *Enabling occupation: An occupational therapy perspective.* Ottawa, ON: Author.

Chambers, A. F. (1999). *What is this thing called science?* (3rd ed.). Indianapolis, IN: Hackett Publishing Company, Inc.

Feins, J. D., & Fosburg, L. B. (1999). Emergency shelter and services: Opening a front door to the continuum of care. In L. Fosburg & D. Dennis (Eds.), *Practical lessons: The 1998 national symposium on homelessness research* (pp. 9:1-36). Washington, DC: U.S Department of Housing and Urban Development and U.S. Department of Health and Human Services.

Fidler, G. S. (2000). Beyond the therapy model: Building our future. *American Journal of Occupational Therapy, 54*, 99-101.

Forsyth, R., & Jarvis, S. (2002). Participation in childhood. *Child: Care, Health and Development, 28*(4), 277-279.

Fosburg, L. B., & Dennis, D. L. (Eds.) (1999). *Practical lessons: The 1998 national symposium on homelessness research.* Washington, DC: U.S. Department of Housing and Urban Development and U.S. Department of Health and Human Services.

Fremstad, S. (2004). *Recent welfare reform research findings: Implications for TANF reauthorization and state TANF policies.* Washington, DC: Center on Budget and Policy Priorities.

Gibson, J. J. (1979). *The ecological approach to visual perception.* Boston: Houghton Mifflin.

Griner, K. R. (in press). Helping the homeless: An occupational therapy perspective. *Occupational Therapy in Mental Health, 22*(1).

Halfon, N., & Hochstein, M. (2002). Life course health development: An integrated framework for developing health, policy, and research. *The Milbank Quarterly, 80*(3), 433-479.

Handler, J. F. (1992). The modern pauper: The homeless in welfare history. In M. J. Robertson & M. Greenblatt (Eds.), *Homelessness: A national perspective* (pp. 35-46). New York: Plenum Press.

Hanson, F. A. (1993). *Testing, testing: Social consequences of the examined life.* Los Angeles: University of California Press.

Huston, A. C. (Ed.) (1991). *Children living in poverty.* New York: Cambridge University Press.

Koegel, P., Burnam, M. A., & Baumohl, J. (1996). The causes of homelessness. In J. Baumohl (Ed.), *Homeless in America* (pp. 24-33). Phoenix, AZ: Oryx Press.

Labonte, R. (1997). Community, community development, and the forming of authentic partnerships. In M. Minkler (Ed.), *Community organizing and community building for health* (pp. 88-102). New Brunswick, NJ: Rutgers University Press.

Law, M. (1991). The environment: A focus for occupational therapy. *Canadian Journal of Occupational Therapy, 58*, 171-179.

Lewis, O. (1966). The culture of poverty. *Scientific America, 215*, 19-25.

Lipman, B. J. (2002). *America's working families and the housing landscape 1997-2001* (Vol. 3). Washington, DC: Center for Housing Policy.

Luthar, S. S. (1999). *Poverty and children's adjustment.* Thousand Oaks, CA: SAGE.

McKinney-Vento Homeless Assistance Act of 1987, 42 U.S.C. §11431 et seq. (2002).

McKnight, J. (1995). *The careless society: Community and its counterfeits*. New York: Basic Books.

McKnight, J. L. (1997). Two tools for well-being: Health systems and communities. In M. Minkler (Ed.), *Community organizing and community building for health* (pp. 20-25). New Brunswick, NJ: Rutgers University Press.

McNichol, E. C. (2005). *State fiscal crisis lingers: Cuts still loom*. Washington, DC: Center on Budget and Policy Priorities.

Merriam-Webster's Collegiate Dictionary (11th ed.) (2003). Springfield, MA: Merriam-Webster.

Merves, E. S. (1992). Homeless women: Beyond the bad lady myth. In M. Robertson & M. Greenblat (Eds.), *Homelessness: A national perspective* (pp. 229-244). New York, NY: Plenum Press.

Moynihan, D. P. (1965). *The Negro family: The case for national action*. Washington, DC: U. S. Department of Labor.

National Low Income Housing Coalition (2005). *Out of reach: 2005*. Retrieved February 10, 2006 from http://www.nlihc.org/oor_current/

Norman, D. A. (1988). *The psychology of everyday things*. New York: Basic Books.

Personal Responsibility and Work Opportunity Reconciliation Act of 1996. 42 U.S.C. §1305 (2002).

Rank, M. R. (1994). *Living on the edge: The realities of welfare in America*. New York: Columbia University Press.

Robertson, M. J., & Greenblatt, M. (1992). Homelessness: A national perspective. In M. Robertson & M. Greenblatt (Eds.), *Homelessness: A national perspective* (pp. 339-349). New York: Plenum Press.

Rog, D. (2002). *Transitioning from homelessness to housing: What works?* Paper presented at the 130th Annual Meeting of American Public Health Association, Philadelphia.

Rog, D. J., & Holupka, C. S. (1999). Reconnecting homeless individuals and families to the community. In L. Fosburg & D. Dennis (Eds.), *Practical lessons: The 1998 national symposium on homelessness research* (pp. 11:11-38). Washington, DC: U. S. Department of Housing and Urban Development.

Rosencheck, R., Bassuk, E., & Salomon, A. (1999). Special populations of homeless Americans. In L. Fosburg & D. Dennis (Eds.) *Practical lessons: The 1998 national symposium on homelessness research* (pp. 2:1-31). Washington, DC: U. S. Department of Housing and Urban Development.

Shinn, M. L., & Weitzman, B. C. (1996). Homeless families are different. In J. Baumohl (Ed.), *Homeless in America* (pp. 109-122). Phoenix, AZ: Oryx.

Smedley, B. D., & Syme, S. L. (Eds.) (2000). *Promoting health: Intervention strategies from social and behavioral research*. Washington, DC: National Academy Press.

Snow, D. A., Anderson, L., & Koegel, P. (1994). Distorting tendencies in research on the homeless. *American Behavioral Scientist, 37*(4), 461-475.

Spaniol, S., & Cattaneo, M. (1997). The power of language in the helping relationship. In L. Spaniol, C. Gagne, & M. Koehler (Eds.), *Psychological and social aspects of psychiatric disability* (pp. 477-484). Boston: Center for Psychiatric Rehabilitation, Sargent College of Health and Rehabilitation Science, Boston University.

U. S. Centers for Disease Control and Prevention (2005a). *Preventing heart disease and stroke*. Retrieved October 1, 2005 from http://www.cdc.gov/nccdphp/bb_heartdisease/index.htm

U. S. Centers for Disease Control and Prevention (2005b). *Stroke fact sheet*. Retrieved October 1, 2005 from http://www.cdc.gov/cvh/library/pdfs/fs_stroke.pdf

U. S. Department of Health and Human Services (1998). *Advisory committee on homeless families: Meeting summary February 27, 1998*. Rockville, MD: Author.

Weinstock-Zlotnick, G., & Hinojosa, J. (2005). Bottom-up or top-down evaluation: Is one better than the other? *American Journal of Occupational Therapy, 58*, 594-599.

Wilson, W. J. (1996). *When work disappears: The world of the new urban poor*. New York: Vintage Books.

Wong, Y. I., Culhane, D. P., & Kuhn, R. (1997). Predictors of exit and re-entry among family shelter users in New York City. *Social Service Review, 71*(3), 441-462.

Wong, Y. I., & Piliavin, I. (1997). A dynamic analysis of homeless-domicile transitions. *Social Problems, 44*(3), 408-423.

World Health Organization (2001). *International classification of functioning, disability, and health*. Geneva, Switzerland: Author.

doi:10.1300/J003v20n03_02

Systems of Care for Persons Who Are Homeless in the United States

Bruce W. Livingston, MPA
Kathleen Swenson Miller, PhD, OTR/L

SUMMARY. Occupational therapists work within various systems that provide services to persons who are homeless, including housing, health care, social service, education, and work programs. This article describes the typologies of homelessness, the continuum of care, trends in service delivery, the federal organization and primary sources of funding for homeless services. It is important for therapists to understand these systems and resources in order to deliver and advocate for effective services for persons who are homeless. doi:10.1300/J003v20n03_03 *[Article copies available for a fee from The Haworth Document Delivery Service: 1-800-HAWORTH. E-mail address: <docdelivery@haworthpress.com> Website: <http://www.HaworthPress.com> © 2006 by The Haworth Press, Inc. All rights reserved.]*

KEYWORDS. Occupational therapy, continuum of care, funding

Bruce W. Livingston is Director of Program Development and Evaluation, The Salvation Army, Eastern Pennsylvania and Delaware Division, Philadelphia, PA.

Kathleen Swenson Miller is Assistant Professor, Department of Occupational Therapy, Jefferson College of Health Professions, Thomas Jefferson University, Philadelphia, PA.

Address correspondence to: Bruce Livingston (E-mail: blivingston@use.salvationarmy.org).

[Haworth co-indexing entry note]: "Systems of Care for Persons Who Are Homeless in the United States." Livingston, Bruce W., and Kathleen Swenson Miller. Co-published simultaneously in *Occupational Therapy in Health Care* (The Haworth Press, Inc.) Vol. 20, No. 3/4, 2006, pp. 31-46; and: *Homelessness in America: Perspectives, Characterizations, and Considerations for Occupational Therapy* (ed: Kathleen Swenson Miller, Georgiana L. Herzberg, and Sharon A. Ray) The Haworth Press, Inc., 2006, pp. 31-46. Single or multiple copies of this article are available for a fee from The Haworth Document Delivery Service [1-800-HAWORTH, 9:00 a.m. - 5:00 p.m. (EST). E-mail address: docdelivery@haworthpress.com].

Available online at http://othc.haworthpress.com
© 2006 by The Haworth Press, Inc. All rights reserved.
doi:10.1300/J003v20n03_03

Homelessness is a complex issue that crosses multiple service systems: housing, health, social services, education, and labor. In the past several years, homeless services have become tailored to subgroups of the homeless population. The purpose of this article is to provide background information on these subgroups of the homeless population as well as on their systems of care, including the continuum of care, program outcome expectations, and common sources of funding for homeless services. How occupational therapists can apply this knowledge of systems to occupational therapy services and research with the homeless population is discussed.

WHO ARE THE HOMELESS?

Most federally funded programs for the homeless use the McKinney-Vento Act definition of homelessness as "an individual who lacks a fixed, regular, and adequate nighttime residence; and a person who has a nighttime residence that is (a) a supervised publicly or privately operated shelter designed to provide temporary living accommodations (including welfare hotels, congregate shelters, and transitional housing for the mentally ill); (b) an institution that provides a temporary residence for individuals intended to be institutionalized; or (c) a public or private place not designed for, nor ordinarily used as, a regular sleeping accommodation for human beings" (McKinney-Vento Act P.L. 100-77, 1987). This federal definition does not include persons who are "doubled up" with family or friends because they have no other place to live, which obscures the true number of persons who are homeless.

It is important to keep in mind the gender breakdown of homelessness. The majority of persons who are homeless are single men (61%); 15% are single women; 15% are women with children; and 9% are adults with another adult (Burt, Aron, Lee, & Valente, 2001). Society tends to be more empathetic to the plight of homeless women with children than to single men.

For people who are homeless, instability is a common denominator: instability of a sense of place; instability of family connections; and instability or lack of housing (Burt et al., 2001). A primary outcome goal for homeless programs is to work towards housing *stability* for their clients, not only to obtain housing. Housing stability implies that persons can obtain housing *plus sustain* their housing by competently carrying out a "home maintainer" role, e.g., paying bills, routine cleaning of their home, getting along with neighbors. Getting access to affordable housing is the goal and primary barrier for most persons who are homeless. For other subgroups of homeless persons, maintaining housing is the greater challenge.

Subgroups of the Homeless Population

Rather than thinking of the homeless population as a homogenous population that is responsive to the same services, it is useful to think of subgroups of persons who are homeless. These subgroups have different characteristics and service needs, identified through Kuhn and Culhane's research (1998). They analyzed administrative data of first time and repeated admissions of emergency shelter users in New York City and Philadelphia over a four-year period of time. The findings suggested that the homeless population consists of three subgroups: the *transitionally* homeless, representing 80% of shelter users; the *episodically* homeless, 10% of shelter users; and the *chronically* homeless, representing 10% of shelter users. What are the characteristics of these three subgroups?

The transitionally homeless. The transitional homeless population has short emergency shelter stays, tends to be younger and is less likely to have mental health, substance abuse or medical problems. These individuals typically use an emergency shelter for a single time, and can fairly quickly resolve the issues that led to their becoming homeless. Examples of persons who are transitionally homeless are those who become homeless because of a house fire or who lose their job and have no savings to pay their rent. The transitionally homeless typically benefit from short emergency shelter stays and assistance to address their immediate personal need. These persons do not typically need long-term support.

Episodically homeless. The second subgroup consists of those *episodically* homeless. This group has had previous admissions to emergency shelter programs. This population is relatively young but is likely to have a mental health, substance abuse, and/or medical problem. Those who are episodically homeless may benefit from moving from an emergency shelter program to a transitional housing program in order to have stable housing while addressing the issues that led to their homelessness. This group is at risk of becoming chronically homeless unless they resolve the issues that led to their trajectory into homelessness.

Chronically homeless. The third subgroup consists of those who are *chronically* homeless. Since 2002, this subgroup has become the priority of federal government homeless initiatives because the *chronically homeless* subgroup uses approximately 50% of homeless shelter funding. This subgroup has multiple emergency shelter admissions, even though they constitute only 10% of emergency shelter users (Kuhn & Culhane,1998). The chronically homeless subgroup tends to be older and have higher levels of mental health, substance abuse, and medical problems. Because of these chronic and disabling health conditions, this subgroup hypothetically is best served by providing permanent supported housing and long-term supported care. Persons who are episodically or chronically homeless are people that occupational therapists have a long professional history of working with to promote optimal self-sufficiency and healthy community engagement.

Persons at Risk for Becoming Transitionally or Chronically Homeless

Episodically homeless persons who have chronic and disabling conditions are logically at risk for becoming transitionally or chronically homeless. Fischer and Breaky (1991) reported that 25% to 33% of the homeless population has a serious mental illness. Thirty-one percent of homeless adults report mental health and substance abuse co-morbidity; 17% reported only substance abuse problems (Burt, 2001). In one county-wide (Alameda County, California) study of homeless persons, 52.4% of persons had a current substance use disorder (Robertson, Zlotnick, & Westefelt, 1997). There are limited prevalence studies of other chronic health problems, learning disabilities or cognitive disabilities that may impact a homeless person's ability to work and potentially maintain stable housing. All of these populations are at risk for having multiple episodes of homelessness because they may have difficulty obtaining or maintaining employment or managing the responsibilities associated with maintaining a household.

The primary, frequently the only, source of income for persons with chronic or disabling conditions with limited job training skills is through Supplemental Security Income (SSI). SSI is a federal income maintenance program, a welcome source of stable income. In 2005, SSI income was approximately $579/month which must cover housing, food and clothing costs; seven states supplement this federal income. Those dependent upon SSI income as their sole income are at an extreme disadvantage in today's housing market (Pitcoff et al., 2005). Only two out of 1000 (.2%) persons who receive SSI stop receiving it (Pasternack, 2003). In many cases, SSI dependence frequently translates to a lifetime of poverty if this is the sole source of income, increasing a person's risk for homelessness.

Housing and Urban Development (HUD) Definitions of Chronic Homelessness and Disabilities

HUD is the primary driver of developing and offering affordable housing for very low income individuals. Of interest to occupational therapists are the HUD operational definitions of chronic homelessness and disabling conditions. As part of an effort to standardize data collected, HUD-funded programs use the following definitions for program reporting purposes. A "chronically homeless" person is defined as "an unaccompanied homeless individual with a disabling condition who has either been continuously homeless for a year or more OR has had at least four (4) episodes of homelessness in the past three (3) years" (HUD, 2004). To be considered chronically homeless, a person must have been on the streets or in an emergency shelter during these stays. HUD defines "disabling condition" as a "diagnosable substance use disorder, serious mental illness, developmental disability, or chronic physical illness or disability, including the co-occurrence of two or more of these conditions. A disabling condition limits an individual's ability to work or perform one or more activities of daily living" (HUD, 2004). Unlike some other federal eligibility criteria guidelines, substance use disorder is considered a disabling condition by HUD.

It is useful to pair this understanding of subgroups of homeless persons with the organization of homeless services. A continuum of services typically exists in local communities to meet the varying needs of subgroups of homeless persons.

CONTINUUM OF SERVICES

A continuum of care utilizes a comprehensive approach to persons who need different types and intensity of services over time, depending upon changing issues.

History of the Continuum of Care Services

The recession in the United States in 1981-82 resulted in a significant increase in demand for emergency shelter and food. Services were primarily crisis and short-term focused, frequently referred to as "three hots (three meals) and a cot (a place to sleep)." In 1987, the Stewart B. McKinney Homeless Assistance Act (Public Law 100-77) became law, later becoming the McKinney-Vento Homeless Assistance Act (CRS Report for Congress, 2005). This legislation drives much of the organizational structure and federal funding for homeless services. By the end of 1980 and early 1990s, some communities began to plan for an organized system of homeless services.

Programs and Services Within the Continuum of Care

Beginning in 1994, HUD required each community that received federal funds to design a continuum of care for their homeless population to meet their community's unique culture and service system; this coherent plan required community-wide service provider cooperation. In creating a continuum of care, each community identifies its service gaps, requests funding to address those gaps, and ranks their proposed projects according to their community's greatest needs. At the local community level, there is significant competition between existing programs and new programs for these federal dollars to address the complex needs of their homeless population.

A community's continuum of care typically includes the following category of services. (1) *Homeless prevention services* include support for problems such as unpaid heating bills, discharge planning from publicly funded institutions such as prisons or rent payment assistance. (2) *Street outreach and assessment* services focus on building trust with persons who are living on the streets, then identification of their personal and health-care needs, and finally referral to appropriate services. (3) *Emergency shelter* programs provide short-term basic food and shelter and referral to necessary services and housing resources. (4) *Transitional housing* programs offer housing and support services for persons who are not ready to manage independent living but need stable housing to address the issues that led to their trajectory into homelessness. Residence in transitional housing programs is typically up to 24 months. Supportive services usually offered by transitional housing programs include case management, drug and alcohol counseling services, education and work training programs, and life skills programs. (5) *Permanent housing* and *permanent supportive housing* is housing designed to meet the long-term needs of homeless individuals and families; at least one person in a family unit must have a disability and meet the federal definition of homelessness (Burt et al., 2001). Homeless services are typically provided by government and not-for-profit organizations, including faith-based groups. Traditionally, persons who become homeless progress step-wise through this continuum of services.

Current Trends in Services

The current federal focus is on chronic homelessness. The current political sense is that chronic homelessness should not be accommodated through emergency shelter programs. There is now an understanding that simply providing emergency shelter care does little to address the complex needs of persons who are chronically homeless. In order to end chronic homelessness, a current trend is to provide *permanent supported housing* to this subgroup. This movement is known as the "housing first" model, typically used with persons who are chronically homeless and have co-morbidities such as serious mental illness and substance abuse (Tsemberis, Gulcur, & Nakae, 2004). The "housing first" model is consumer-driven where individuals are provided housing along with support services if the consumer feels he can manage a less supervised living circumstance than is typically provided in transitional housing. The "housing first" model does *not* require someone to be "substance free" or compliant with a mental health program in order to get his or her own housing. Support services are offered, but the consumer has the right to refuse them. The assumption of a "housing first" model is that stable housing is an immediate need and that people prefer to live in their own place rather than in forms of congregate housing that have institutional policies. Tsemberis, Gulcur and Nakae's research (2004) indicated that individuals who participated in a "housing first" program obtained housing earlier, remained stably housed, and had equivalent substance use and psychiatric symptoms as persons who participated in a transitional congregate living program.

This emphasis on chronic homelessness is controversial. Some within the homeless advocacy community feel that this focus has limited the attention and financial resources for prevention of homelessness, addressing the needs of homeless families, and addressing the core issues of poverty and affordable housing (National Coalition for the Homeless, 2005).

Coordination of Systems of Care

At the federal level, the Interagency Council on Homelessness coordinates the efforts of 18 federal agencies that touch the lives of persons who are homeless (Sullivan, 2002). At the local level, coordination of efforts exists between programs that provide homeless services, especially housing services. A continuum of care at the local level requires a careful balance of emergency, transitional, permanent housing, and support services.

Recent Emphasis on Encouraging Enrollment in Mainstream Benefits

In 2001, Congress mandated programs that serve the homeless to integrate their programs with "mainstream" programs (http://www.nlchp.org/). Mainstream programs include entitlement programs such as food stamps, government-funded health care programs, and "One Stop Shopping" employment services. Persons who are homeless are frequently unable to access these entitlement programs due to lack of knowledge about them, how to access them, or having a permanent address to obtain them. Providing access to these mainstream services gives more resources to a person who is homeless, potentially reducing the number of risk factors for repeated shelter admissions. For example, if a person gets health insurance through mainstream benefits, he could hypothetically obtain health maintenance treatment for a health condition such as diabetes. This health care may enable this person to work, avoiding emergency hospitalizations. Thus, he may have a source of income to pay his rent, preventing an episode of homelessness.

Homeless Management Information System (HMIS)

In an effort to guide a community's planning process, Congress has directed jurisdictions to collect an array of data on their community's homeless population and services, including: unduplicated counts of the number of people homeless, use of services, and the effectiveness of the local homeless assistance systems. Local jurisdictions are gradually implementing use of a database to collect common information. This system is known as the Homeless Management Information System (HUD, 2005).

Aside from federal outcome reporting requirements, each program's funding source typically requires reporting on the program's effectiveness. The program's outcomes are usually measured against federal outcome requirements as well as individual program goals. The program's goals are usually dependent upon the program's placement in the continuum of care.

It is important for occupational therapists to understand a program's goals and how they are measured, in order to intersect the therapist's intervention goals with the program goals. For example, typical program outcomes expected from HUD-funded transitional and permanent housing programs include: achieve residential stability; increase work skills and/or income; and obtain greater self-determination. These outcome goals are designed to aid homeless persons to become optimally self-sufficient. For an occupational therapist working within a transitional housing program, intersecting therapy goals may include goals that address developing home maintainer roles, productivity goals or, perhaps, money management.

Occupational therapists who work within homeless programs must be mindful of the overall program goals, and can be strong contributors to building positive program outcomes. Another contribution that an occupational therapist can make is to assist in the development of realistic program goals, especially for programs that serve largely episodically and chronically homeless populations.

GOVERNMENT PROGRAMS FOR HOMELESS SERVICES

Table 1 describes the major government programs and sources of funding of services for persons who are homeless.

Occupational therapists can consider how to intersect their knowledge and skill sets with this array of services by understanding the various contexts in which homeless services are or could be delivered.

THE SERVICE PROVIDERS WITHIN THE SERVICE SYSTEM

Service providers have been the traditional link between the homeless system of services and persons who are homeless. Liebow (1993) described the range of service providers he observed during his four years as a participant observer while working with several shelters. The milieu of the shelters ranged from laissez-faire to democratically run to highly regimented, autocratic environments. The staff perceptions of their jobs ranged from that of a professional purpose to "change the women" in order to assist them out of homelessness to that of providing a safe refuge for life's basic necessities of food and shelter. Staff and volunteer attitudes towards the people they served ranged from perceptions of "freeloaders" and "undeserving" to "that could be me." These staff attitudes impacted staff behavior which ranged from acts of disrespect to acts of kindness and generosity. Liebow talked about the attitude, "you mustn't make things too easy for them" that he repeatedly observed play out in staff behavior

TABLE 1. Federal Programs Related to Homelessness

Program Name	Participant Eligibility	Services	Funding Source Plus Where to Find Information
Housing and Food			
Emergency Food and Shelter Program (EFSP)	Local EFSP Boards determine participant eligibility. Any criteria used must provide for assistance to needy individuals without discrimination (age, race, sex, religion, national origin, disability, economic status, or sexual orientation)	• Food • Lodging in a shelter or hotel • One month's rent or mortgage payment • One month's utility bill • Minor repairs for food facilities or shelters • Equipment to feed or shelter people	Federal Emergency Management Agency (FEMA) *http://www.fema.gov/rrr/efs.shtm* United Way of America (National Board) *http://www.efsp.unitedway.org/efsp/pages/about.htm* Local United Way
Housing			
Emergency Shelter Grant (ESG)	• Individuals meeting the federal definition of being homeless • Individuals at risk of becoming homeless; must be able to resume rent/utility payments within a reasonable period of time	• Funding for emergency shelter and essential supportive services (employment, health, drug abuse, and/or education) • Homeless prevention including financial assistance for rent and utilities • Federal dollars matched one for one with local resources	U.S. Department of Housing and Urban Development (HUD) *http://www.hud.gov/offices/cpd/homeless/library/esg/esgdeskguide/index.cfm* State, county or city governments
Supportive Housing Program –Supportive Services Only (SHP-SSO)	Individuals meeting the federal definition of being homeless	• Homeless outreach, case management, life skills education, alcohol and drug abuse services, mental health services, other health care services, education, housing placement, employment assistance, child care, transportation, legal, and other assistance	U.S. Department of Housing and Urban Development (HUD) *http://www.hud.gov/offices/cpd/homeless/library/shp/shpdeskguide/index.cfm* State, regional, county, or city governments
Supportive Housing Program –Transitional Housing	• Individuals meeting the federal definition of being homeless • Residency in an emergency shelter	• Transitional housing for up to 24 months with supportive social services • Supportive service supports • Settings include both single-site facilities (single room occupancy SRO and apartments and scattered-site apartments and houses)	U.S. Department of Housing and Urban Development (HUD) *http://www.hud.gov/offices/cpd/homeless/library/shp/shpdeskguide/index.cfm* State, regional, county, or city governments
Supportive Housing Program –Permanent Housing for Persons with Disabilities	• Individuals meeting the federal definition of being homeless • At least one member of the household must have a disability verified in writing from a qualified source	• Long-term, community-based housing with supportive services for persons with disabilities • Enables special needs populations to live as independently as possible • Settings include both single-site facilities (single room occupancy SRO and apartments and scattered-site apartments and houses) • Supportive services include one or more of those noted for SSO programs	U.S. Department of Housing and Urban Development (HUD) *http://www.hud.gov/offices/cpd/homeless/library/shp/shpdeskguide/index.cfm* State, regional, county, or city governments

Program Name	Participant Eligibility	Services	Funding Source Plus Where to Find Information
Housing (continued)			
Supportive Housing Program –Safe Haven	Homeless individuals who have a serious mental illness, live on the street and have been unable or unwilling to participate in housing or supportive services	• Supportive housing for this hard-to-reach population • Services include intensive outreach and assessment, 24-hour program residence for an unspecified amount of time in private or semi-private accommodations with access to supportive services such as case management and mental health services • "Low-demand" program meaning that participants are not required to utilize supportive services	U.S. Department of Housing and Urban Development (HUD) *http://www.hud.gov/offices/cpd/homeless/library/shp/shpdeskguide/index.cfm* State, regional, county, or city governments
Shelter Plus Care (S+C)	Homeless and disabled At least one adult member of a household must be disabled	• Rental assistance that local programs must match with an equal value of supportive services appropriate to the target population • Housing affordability through using grant funds to pay the difference between actual rent for a unit and 30 percent of the participant's income • Supportive services same as noted above for SHP-SSO	U.S. Department of Housing and Urban Development (HUD) *http://www.hud.gov/offices/cpd/homeless/library/spc/resourcemanual/index.cfm* State, regional, county, or city governments
Single Room Occupancy (SRO)	Individuals meeting the federal definition of being homeless	• Rental assistance in renovated SRO dwellings • SRO housing for one person occupancy • Individual units may contain kitchens and/or bathrooms or shared facilities • Rental assistance covers difference between a portion of the tenant's income (normally 30%) and the unit's rent, which must be within the local or regional fair market rent (FMR) established by HUD	U.S. Department of Housing and Urban Development (HUD) *http://www.hud.gov/offices/cpd/homeless/programs/sro/index.cfm* State, regional, county, or city governments
Title V Program	Individuals meeting the federal definition of being homeless	• Surplus federal property available to States, local governments, and non-profit organizations • Space can be used to provide shelter and/or support services • No funding for renovation of space	U.S. Department of Housing and Urban Development (HUD) *http://www.hud.gov/offices/cpd/homeless/programs/t5/index.cfm* U.S. Department of Health and Human Services manages the application process
Housing Choice Vouchers (Section 8 Program)	Individuals and families with very low incomes, below 50% of the median household income for the local or regional area	• Very low-income families can choose to lease safe, decent, and affordable privately owned rental housing • Local public housing authority pays landlords the difference between 30% of household income and the fair market rent for that area	U.S. Department of Housing and Urban Development (HUD) *http://www.hud.gov/offices/pih/programs/hcv/index.cfm* Local Public Housing Authority

TABLE 1 (continued)

Program Name	Participant Eligibility	Services	Funding Source Plus Where to Find Information
Housing (continued)			
HOPWA (Housing Opportunities for People with AIDS)	Low-income persons medically diagnosed with HIV/AIDS and their families	• Housing assistance and related supportive services • Rehabilitation, or new construction of housing units; facility operation costs; rental assistance; and short-term payments to prevent homelessness • Health care, mental health, substance abuse, nutritional services, case management, & daily living assistance	U.S. Department of Housing and Urban Development (HUD) *http://www.hud.gov/offices/cpd/aidshousing/programs/index.cfm*
The Low Income Housing Tax Credit (LIHTC) Program	Households with an initial qualifying income at or below 60% of the area median income (AMI)	Equity capital for the construction and rehabilitation of affordable rental housing	U.S. Department of Housing and Urban Development (HUD) *http://www.hud.gov/offices/cpd/affordablehousing/training/lihtc/index.cfm*
HOME Program	Households with an income at or below 60% of the area median income (AMI)	• Incentives to develop and support affordable rental housing and homeownership affordability • HOME funds can assist renters and new homebuyers	U.S. Department of Housing and Urban Development (HUD) *http://www.hud.gov/offices/cpd/affordablehousing/index.cfm*
Multi-Purpose			
Community Development Block Grant (CDBG)	• 51% of the households served by an activity or program must have low-to-moderate income, meaning less than 80% of the area median income (AMI) • In 2005, the national family median income was $58,000. HUD annually determines median income for each area annually	• Annual formula grants to entitled cities, urban counties and states to develop viable urban communities by providing decent housing and a suitable living environment, and by expanding economic opportunities, mainly for low- and moderate-income persons • Affordable housing and community infrastructure development	U.S. Department of Housing and Urban Development (HUD) *http://www.hud.gov/offices/cpd/communitydevelopment/programs/entitlement/index.cfm* State, county, or city governments
Homeless Veterans Reintegration Project	Veterans of the United States military who are homeless	• Employment and training services needed to reenter the labor market, e.g., job counseling, resume preparation, skills assessment, job development and placement • Supportive services such as clothing, shelter, referral to medical or substance abuse treatment, and transportation assistance	U.S. Department of Labor *http://www.dol.gov/vets/programs/fact/Homeless_ veterans_fs04.htm*
Homeless Providers Grant and Per Diem Program	Veterans of the United States military who are homeless	• Provides supportive housing and/ or supportive services • Services include supportive housing for up to 24 months and service centers offering case management, crisis intervention, and counseling	Department of Veterans Affairs *http://www1.va.gov/homeless/page.cfm?pg=3*

Program Name	Participant Eligibility	Services	Funding Source Plus Where to Find Information
Health			
Healthcare for the Homeless (HCH)	An individual or family who lacks housing including those whose primary residence at night is a supervised emergency shelter or transitional housing	• Only federal program with responsibility for addressing the primary care needs of the homeless • Program provides community-based primary and emergency care, mental health, and substance abuse services • Outreach to difficult-to-place homeless persons is a program emphasis	U.S. Department of Health and Human Services, Health Resources and Services Administration, Bureau of Primary Health Care *http://bphc.hrsa.gov/hchirc/about/comp_response.htm*
Projects for Assistance in Transition from Homelessness (PATH)	Persons at risk for becoming homeless who have serious mental illness and homeless persons with serious mental illnesses	• Community-based services for those homeless or at risk of becoming homeless and who have serious mental illnesses and / or co-occurring substance abuse disorders • Services including outreach, screening, assessment, case management, mental health and substance abuse treatment, and other supportive services	U.S. Department of Health and Human Services, Substance Abuse and Mental Health Services Administration, The Center for Mental Health Services *http://pathprogram.samhsa.gov/about/overview.asp*
Addiction Treatment for the Homeless	Homeless persons with substance abuse concerns	• Enables communities to enhance drug and alcohol treatment systems for homeless individuals with substance abuse disorders or with co-occurring substance abuse and mental disorders • Addresses the need to link D & A services with housing, and to secure and maintain housing for homeless persons with substance abuse problems	U.S. Department of Health and Human Services, Substance Abuse and Mental Health Services Administration *http://www.samhsa.gov/Matrix/programs_homeless2.aspx*
Preventive Health Block Grant	Underserved populations	• Supports clinical services, preventive screening, laboratory support, outbreak control, workforce training, public education, data surveillance, and program evaluation targeting such health problems as cardiovascular disease, cancer, diabetes, emergency medical services, injury and violence prevention, infectious disease, environmental health, community fluoridation, and sex offenses • Emphasis placed on adolescents, communities with little or poor health care services, and disadvantaged populations	U.S. Department of Health and Human Services, Center for Disease Control and Prevention *http://www.cdc.gov/nccdphp/blockgrant/faqs.htm*
Education			
Education for Homeless Children and Youth	Children and youth who lack a fixed, regular, and adequate nighttime residence are considered homeless	• Addresses problems that homeless children and youth face in enrolling, attending, and succeeding in school • Every Local Education Agency required to designate a local liaison serving as the primary contact between homeless families and school staff. Liaison coordinates services so that children can succeed academically	U.S. Department of Education *http://www.ed.gov/programs/homeless/guidance.pdf* State departments of education and/or local school districts

TABLE 1 (continued)

Program Name	Participant Eligibility	Services	Funding Source Plus Where to Find Information
Employment			
Workforce Investment Act (WIA)	Universal access for adults; intensive and specialized services for laid-off workers and youth	• National infrastructure for a coordinated system to provide comprehensive employment and training services and information • One-Stop Career Centers	U.S. Department of Labor *http://www.doleta.gov/usworkforce/wia.cfm* Local Workforce Investment Board
Social Services			
Social Services Block Grant		• Allocates funds to States to support social service programs for adults and children • Services directed toward, among others, to achieving or maintaining self-sufficiency • Case management, child day care, life skills education, employment services, housing counseling, transition from homelessness to independent living, information and referral, legal services, and substance abuse services	U.S. Department of Health and Human Services, Administration for Children and Families *http://www.acf.hhs.gov/programs/ocs/ssbg/*

and homeless policy, reflected in organizational and policy roadblocks for homeless persons.

Societal values seem to be ambiguously conflicted between a general societal attitude that poor people are not deserving of public support in contrast to a fear of providing too much support, resulting in dependency on that support. Finlayson, Baker, Rodman, and Herzberg (2002) discovered that shelter residents' goals differed from staff goals for the residents, reflecting some of these societal conflicts. The authors concluded that one important role for therapists is to bridge differences between residents and staff perceptions of residents' needs which affect goal setting. The occupational therapist's services may include direct evaluation and intervention services to persons who are homeless, but also as a consultant and educator to program staff.

RELATION OF OCCUPATIONAL THERAPY TO SYSTEMS OF CARE

Occupational therapists can and do work in the full array of programs that provide services to persons who are homeless. Occupational therapists have particularly useful skills to help the *episodically homeless* and *chronically homeless* populations, who typically have chronic health conditions and disabilities. For persons who are episodically homeless in the emergency shelter system, occupational therapists may assist in the development of realistic transitional planning, especially if an individual has a chronic health condition or disabling condition. Occupational therapists can provide important supportive services in transitional housing or permanent supportive housing programs, where housing stability is achieved. Occupational therapists have unique educational backgrounds in understanding the role of occupational participation and its relationship to disability and prevention of disability. The Occupational Therapy Practice Framework (American Occupational Therapy Association, 2002) provides a lens for understanding the complex issues that impact daily functioning in occupational performance areas such as work or home maintenance skills. This knowledge base can be useful in working directly with persons who are homeless, consulting with program staff, or with program development and evaluation to meet the unique needs of subgroups of homeless persons.

Understanding the systems of care can guide the therapist's focus for assessment, intervention, and research. Occupational therapists must consider variables such as chronic homelessness and disability, as well as the point in the continuum of care where participants receive services. It is important for occupational therapists to understand the complex issues of homelessness and the systems of care in order to assist homeless persons to rebuild their lives or live a meaningful life.

REFERENCES

American Occupational Therapy Association (2002). Occupational therapy practice framework: Domain and process. *American Journal of Occupational Therapy, 56*, 609-639.

Burt, M.R. (September 2001). What will it take to end homelessness? Washington, DC: Urban Institute Press. Retrieved December 2, 2005 from http://www.urban.org/uploadedPDF/end_homelessness.pdf

Burt, M., Aron, L.Y., Lee, E., & Valente, J. (2001). *Helping America's homeless: Emergency shelter or affordable housing?* Washington, DC: Urban Institute Press.

Finlayson, M., Baker, M., Rodman, L., & Herzberg, G. (2002). The process and outcomes of a multimethod needs assessment at a homeless shelter. *American Journal of Occupational Therapy, 56*, 313-321.

Fischer, P.J., & Breaky, W.R. (1991). The epidemiology of alcohol, drug, and mental disorders among homeless persons. *American Psychology, 46*, 1115-1128.

Kuhn, R., & Culhane, D. (1998). Applying cluster analysis to test a typology of homelessness by pattern of shelter utilization: Results from the analysis of administrative data. *American Journal of Community Psychology, 26*, 207-232.

Liebow, E. (1993). *Tell them who I am: The lives of homeless women*. New York, NY: Penguin Books.

National Coalition for the Homeless. Questions and answers about the chronic homelessness initiative. Retrieved February 26, 2006, from http://www.nationalhomeless.org/publications/chronic/chronicqanda.html

Pasternack, R. (2003, April 3). Highlights of "No child left behind & special education: The view from Washington." Assistant Secretary for Special Education & Rehabiliation Services, U.S. Dept. of Education. Retrieved September 30, 2005 from http://www.ers.princeton.edu/summary.pdf

Pitcoff, W., Pelletiere, D., Crowley, S., Treskon, M., & Dolbeare, C.N. (2004). Out of reach, 2005. National Low Income Housing Coalition. Retrieved February 16, 2006 from http://www.nlihc.org/oor2005

Robertson, M.J., Zlotnick, C., & Westefelt, A. (1997). Drug use disorders and treatment contact among homeless adults in Alameda County, California. *American Journal of Public Health, 87,* 221-228.

Sullivan, B. (2002, July 19). Martinex outlines Bush administration strategy to combat chronic homelessness. U.S. Department of Housing and Urban Development's Homes and Communities. Retrieved September 19, 2005 from www.hud.gov/news/release.cfm?CONTENT=PR02-080.cfm.

Tsemberis, S., Guleur, L., & Nakae, M. (2004). Housing first, consumer choice, and harm reduction for homeless individuals with a dual diagnosis. *American Journal of Public Health, 94,* 651-656.

U.S. Department of Housing and Urban Development (HUD) (October 31, 2005). Homeless management information strategies. Retrieved December 2, 2005 from http://www.hud.gov/offices/cpd/homeless/hmis/

U.S. Department of Housing and Urban Development (HUD) (2004, February). Determining, documenting, and verifying participant eligibility in the Supportive Housing Program. Retrieved February 22, 2006, from http://www.hud.gov/local/wi/working/localpo/cpd/ta.pdf

doi:10.1300/J003v20n03_03

Occupational Concerns of Women Who Are Homeless and Have Children: An Occupational Justice Critique

Betsy VanLeit, PhD, OTR/L, FAOTA
Rebecca Starrett, MOT, OTR/L
Terry K. Crowe, PhD, OTR/L, FAOTA

Betsy VanLeit is Assistant Professor, Occupational Therapy Graduate Program, University of New Mexico. Rebecca Starrett is Occupational Therapist, Albuquerque Public Schools, Albuquerque, NM. Terry K. Crowe is Professor and Director, Occupational Therapy Graduate Program, University of New Mexico.

Address correspondence to: Terry K. Crowe, Occupational Therapy Graduate Program, Health Sciences Center, MSC09 5240, 1 University of New Mexico, Albuquerque, NM 87131(E-mail: tkcrowe@salud.unm.edu).

The authors wish to thank Christine Kroening, MOT, OTR/L, for her active involvement in developing protocols and interviewing women for this project. In addition, a heartfelt thanks goes to the women who agreed to the interviews and spent time telling us about their experiences with being homeless and caring for children.

[Haworth co-indexing entry note]: "Occupational Concerns of Women Who Are Homeless and Have Children: An Occupational Justice Critique." VanLeit, Betsy, Rebecca Starrett, and Terry K. Crowe. Co-published simultaneously in *Occupational Therapy in Health Care* (The Haworth Press, Inc.) Vol. 20, No. 3/4, 2006, pp. 47-62; and: *Homelessness in America: Perspectives, Characterizations, and Considerations for Occupational Therapy* (ed: Kathleen Swenson Miller, Georgiana L. Herzberg, and Sharon A. Ray) The Haworth Press, Inc., 2006, pp. 47-62. Single or multiple copies of this article are available for a fee from The Haworth Document Delivery Service [1-800-HAWORTH, 9:00 a.m. - 5:00 p.m. (EST). E-mail address: docdelivery@haworthpress.com].

Available online at http://othc.haworthpress.com
© 2006 by The Haworth Press, Inc. All rights reserved.
doi:10.1300/J003v20n03_04

SUMMARY. The purpose of this exploratory study was to describe the occupational goals and concerns of women who are homeless with children. Twenty-seven women with children living in homeless shelters completed interviews using the Canadian Occupational Performance Measure (COPM). Occupational issues and concerns were identified for each participant, and then they were pooled. A total of 169 occupational concerns were described and analyzed. The most common occupational issues identified by participants concerned finances, employment, education, transportation, housing, time for self, personal appearance, home management, and parenting. Analysis of identified occupational concerns suggests that the homeless women with children experienced a range of institutional and social barriers to occupational participation: essentially a form of occupational injustice. This study raises questions concerning the most effective roles for occupational therapists to facilitate empowerment so that women who are homeless may fully participate in the communities where they live. doi:10.1300/J003v20n03_04 *[Article copies available for a fee from The Haworth Document Delivery Service: 1-800-HAWORTH. E-mail address: <docdelivery@haworthpress.com> Website: <http://www.HaworthPress.com>* *© 2006 by The Haworth Press, Inc. All rights reserved.]*

KEYWORDS. Occupational therapy, participation, social justice

INTRODUCTION

Skid row, Bowery bum . . . once upon a time these were the places and names symbolic of homelessness in the United States. During the 1950s, women accounted for only 3% of the homeless population (Rossi, 1990). Until the 1970s most of the homeless population in the United States were transient men who followed construction and industrial development across the country and then returned to low-rent sections of cities when work was scarce (Burt, Aron, Lee, & Valente, 2001). But all of that started changing by the 1970s when families began to appear in shelters and organizations that had previously served single adults. By the 1980s, families with children emerged as one of the fastest growing and largest segments of the homeless population (Nunez & Fox, 1999; Bassuk et al., 1996). Toward the late 1990s, women and single mothers with children accounted for 40% of people who were homeless (U.S. Conference of Mayors, 2001), and 85% of homeless families were headed by single women (Roth & Fox, 1990). Factors associated with these demographic changes include welfare reforms, domestic violence, drug abuse, and the demise of low-income housing (Bassuk et al., 1997).

In recent years, occupational therapists have worked with people who are homeless (Finlayson, Baker, Rodman, & Herzberg, 2002; Herzberg & Finlayson, 2001; Schultz-Krohn, 2004; Kavanagh & Fares, 1995; Mitchell & Jones, 1997), including subpopulations of homeless women with post-traumatic stress disorder (Davis & Kutter, 1998) and homeless men and women in emergency shelters (Tryssenaar, Jones, & Lee, 1999). Several authors have described introducing occupational therapy students to fieldwork with homeless individuals (Heubner & Tryssenaar, 1996; Finlayson, Baker, Rodman, & Herzberg, 2002; Drake, 1992).

Since women have become a dominant subgroup of the homeless population, this study focused on women who are homeless and have children. We wanted to describe the women's experience in terms of the impact of homelessness on perceptions of occupational performance and participation. Ultimately, the intent is to help clarify an appropriate framework for occupational therapy practitioners to work with homeless populations that enhances client-centered practice and occupational participation outcomes.

METHODS

Participants

Twenty-seven women who were homeless and had children living with them were recruited to participate in the study. Homelessness was defined as having no stable residence for at least one week. Women who met study inclusion criteria were 18 years or older, had at least one of their children living with them, spoke and understood English, were living in a temporary (shelter) housing arrangement, and voluntarily agreed to participate in the study. The study took place in a large southwestern city in the United States.

Four (15%) of the participants were recruited through a local homeless shelter for women and children. The shelter has a capacity of 15 women plus 10 children, and permits them to stay for a maximum of three weeks. A large percentage of women who come to stay at this shelter have personal histories of domestic violence. During their time at the shelter, the women are assisted by a case manager.

Twenty-three (85%) of the women were residing in a women's shelter that specifically provided temporary housing to women and their children who are survivors of domestic violence. The residents can stay in this shelter for a maximum of 90 days. The shelter has a capacity of 100 women and their children.

Participant demographics are described in Tables 1 and 2. Table 1 includes information on the women's age, ethnicity, grade completed in

TABLE 1. Participant Demographics (n = 27 women)

Characteristic	n	(%)
Age in Years		
18-20	1	(3)
21-25	4	(15)
26-30	5	(19)
	10	(37)
36-40	3	(11)
41-45	4	(15)
Ethnicity		
White/Non-Hispanic	14	(52)
Hispanic	12	(44)
Native American	4	(15)
African American	1	(4)
Other	2	(7)
Level of Education		
Did not complete high school	14	(52)
Completed high school	9	(33)
Completed some college	4	(15)
Number of Children with Women		
1	9	(33)
2	10	(37)
3	3	(11)
4	5	(19)
Age of Children in Years (n = 58 children)		
0-2	11	(19)
3-5	11	(19)
6-8	11	(19)
9-11	13	(22)
12-14	7	(12)
15-18	4	(7)
Over 18	1	(2)
Partner Status		
Identified self as single parent	23	(85)
Identified having a partner	4	(15)

TABLE 2. Participant Housing and Economic Characteristics (n = 27 women)

Characteristic	n	(%)
Type of Housing Lived in Prior to Becoming Homeless		
Apartment	11	(40)
House	13	(48)
Mobile Home	1	(4)
Hotel	1	(4)
None identified	1	(4)
Monthly Income (current)		
None	2	(7)
$1-$200	4	(15)
$201-$500	10	(38)
$501-$800	7	(26)
Over $800	3	(11)
Preferred not to say	1	(3)
Reported Length of Time at Current Location		
Less than 2 weeks	8	(29)
3-4 weeks	3	(11)
1-3 months	9	(34)
Unsure	7	(26)
Length of Time Homeless in Lifetime		
1-4 weeks	13	(49)
1-3 months	5	(19)
3-6 months	3	(10)
6 months-1 year	1	(4)
1 to 2 years	2	(7)
Over 2 years	3	(11)

school, number of children living with them, and partner status. Table 2 describes the participants' status in terms of prior housing, economic status, and amount of time spent being homeless.

Instrument

We used the *Canadian Occupational Performance Measure[COPM]* (Law et al., 1998) as our interview tool. Since its inception over a decade ago, the COPM has been used and evaluated widely in research, practice and education (see for example McColl et al., 1999; Ripat, Etcheverry, Cooper, & Tate, 2001; Toomey, Nicholson, & Carswell, 1995). The COPM's psychometric properties have been evaluated favorably for content, criterion and construct validity (Chan & Lee, 1997; McColl et al., 1999).

Essentially the COPM provided a semi-structured interview format to ask the women about their occupational concerns and issues as well as their perceptions of their current occupational performance and satisfaction. The interview format divides occupational issues into the areas of "Self-Care," "Productivity" and "Leisure," areas consistent with occupational performance areas in the Canadian Model of Occupational Performance [CMOP] (Canadian Association of Occupational Therapists, 1997), and in fact the COPM was designed as an assessment tool that could be used with the CMOP as a guiding model. The CMOP describes the factors that are important to creation of occupation, and its sister model, the Person-Environment-Occupational Model (PEO) emphasizes attention to the fit of the component parts (person, occupation and environment) to optimal occupational performance (Canadian Association of Occupational Therapists, 1997).

Procedures

After receiving University of New Mexico Human Research Review Committee approval, an experienced occupational therapist and researcher (the first author) trained two researchers (occupational therapy graduate students) to collect participant data. After successful pilot testing and finalization of procedural reliability, participants were recruited from the two shelters. The first author observed every fifth interview to assure that the data collectors continued to follow consistent interview procedures throughout the study.

With guidance from the shelter managers, shelter staff and case managers recruited the women, arranged interview times, provided private interview space for the researchers, and introduced the researchers to the women who agreed to participate. After establishing initial rapport, the researchers introduced the consent form which was then read, discussed and signed before initiating the interview. In addition to gathering demographic data and completing the COPM, the researchers also collected time use data for each participant. The results of the time use component of the investigation are reported elsewhere (Kroening, 2002). Each interview was audiotaped and researchers took written notes as well, including actual quotes from the women while filling out the COPM form. Interviews lasted from one to two hours, and after completion, each participant was given a gift certificate to thank her for her time.

Data Analysis

Data were analyzed using descriptive statistics. For demographic data we determined frequencies. For COPM occupational concerns, we listed all of the occupational concerns and then grouped similar ones together (e.g., all occupational concerns about needing to obtain employment were counted together). This allowed us to then characterize types of occupational concerns, as well as frequencies of types of concerns. We also qualitatively used actual quotes from participants to better illustrate occupational concerns.

RESULTS

Participants identified multiple occupational concerns for a pooled total of 169 issues. Table 3 lists the occupational concerns identified by the women in descending order of frequency.

In addition to identifying occupational issues, participants were asked to rate them for importance on a scale of 1-10 (1 being unimportant and 10 being extremely important). The mean rating was 8.62, indicating overall high importance of occupational concerns that were listed.

The greatest number of concerns listed had to do with inadequate finances. The women described issues that ranged from worrying about not having enough money to pay for living expenses, to concerns about saving money for the future, to actually obtaining control over family finances at all (some women were currently separated from husbands or partners who had control over financial resources).

The next most common concern revolved around employment. Issues included being unemployed, being underemployed, needing a job that allowed for flexible scheduling, and having work that paid adequately to support a family. One woman stated: "It's hard for me to get a job, but I want to be in the right job, in the right place."

Educational concerns came next in order of frequency. Women identified concerns about their lack of education, and this was often reported in association with their lack of adequate employment. In the words of one woman: "Staying in school is my way out of this life . . ."

TABLE 3. Identified COPM Concerns (n = 169)

Type of Concern	n
Finances	18
Employment	16
Education	15
Transportation	15
Housing	14
Time for Self	13
Personal Appearance	10
Home Management	10
Care of Children/Parenting	10
Spending more Time with Children	9
Family/Friend Support	7
Safety	7
Childcare (by other Adults)	6
Time in Community with Children	5
Sobriety	5
Spirituality	4
Issues with Shelter Rules/Staff	2
Travel/Vacation	1
Sleep	1

Transportation concerns were also common as many of the participants in the study did not own their own vehicle or have access to a car. Many women reported needing a vehicle to go to work, school or appointments, and they perceived public transportation as inadequate (several women stated that it could take hours to accomplish one appointment across town using the bus).

Not surprisingly, quite a few women voiced concerns about housing. However, it is interesting that this was not identified more often given that all of the women were currently homeless. The words: "I'd like to have a place of my own" were spoken by a number of women. They expressed frustration with the paucity of assistance available to help them obtain housing, and with the general dearth of affordable places to live that were big enough for a family and in a safe part of town.

Lack of time for self was the next most commonly identified occupational concern, followed by the related issue of having time and resources to attend to personal appearance. Participants spoke about how difficult it was to follow a "normal" routine while homeless, and that they never were alone. Women spoke about the unmet need to exercise, relax, read, sleep or just be alone in order to respond more effectively to the changes and stresses in their lives. In terms of personal appearance, one woman stated: "When you're here (the shelter) you don't come with make up and curling irons . . . your self-esteem is down . . . and when you can't fix your hair, fix your face, fix your nails, it's hard. If you can't make yourself look nice, it gets you down."

The next categories of occupational concerns listed had to do with home management, with taking care of their children, with spending more time with their children, and with safety. Home management issues tended to revolve around lack of a stable place and routines (e.g., not being able to do laundry regularly, or not being able to obtain nutritious meals for the family). Concerns about caring for children (also described as parenting by a few women) typically had to do with wanting to raise their children well, and provide for their children. In the words of one participant: "I want to be as good a parent as I can be, maybe I can take parenting classes through the shelter." Another stated: "Since I've been here [the shelter] my mind is so boggled. It is like I'm not really paying attention to my kids . . . I'm listening to what they are saying but my mind is really set somewhere else, so it's not on them like it should be. Now it's just half attention because I'm thinking, what am I going to do tomorrow for food . . . ." Sometimes the women described a simple desire to spend more quality time with their children. Closely related was the occupational concern about safety. As stated by one participant: "I want to be able to take care of my kids. I want us to be safe; I don't want us to be out there and scared about everything."

Next in frequency, participants talked about the importance of relationships with family and friends. Several stated that they were "entirely alone," without support from other adults. Several had recently (and suddenly) left relationships with husbands or boyfriends that had ended violently. Other occupational concerns were identified, but less frequently (from 1-5 times). These are listed at the bottom of Table 3.

DISCUSSION

Limitations

This study described the occupational concerns of only 27 homeless women with children from two shelters in one urban area of the southwestern United States. They may be different from homeless women in other geographical regions or rural areas of the country.

Many of the women had only become homeless recently and/or had been homeless for a brief period of time. The interviewers did not ask the women to describe specifically what life circumstances brought them to the shelter. However, both shelters were known to provide assistance to women who experienced domestic abuse (often the women were in the process of leaving an abusive partner). Thus, the sample in this study may only represent a particular subset of women who are temporarily homeless due to challenging family circumstances.

Finally, the researchers met only once with each participant, and used a semi-structured interview tool to obtain information. Possibly the women did not feel comfortable sharing their concerns openly and honestly with researchers they had just met. A series of interviews and/or interactions with the participants may have raised issues and concerns that did not surface in this study.

Homelessness, Marginalization and Occupational Justice

A main theme identified through interviews in a prior study of men and women who were homeless (Tryssenaar, Jones, & Lee, 1999) was: "We want what everyone wants." That line could easily apply to the current study as well. Wanting a stable place to live, a way to get around town, employment that pays the bills, and a sense of safety in daily life certainly resonate as goals that any of us might wish for in their absence. Similarly, Banyard and Graham-Bermann (1995) interviewed 64 women in temporary shelters and found the wish for a better life for themselves and their children as a top priority. These women felt that going back to school or getting job training would be critical to successfully accomplishing this priority. In a study of 109 Black and Hispanic women who were homeless and had addictions, Nyamathi and Flaskerud (1992) described how the absence of financial security, temporary living situations, and limited social support left them in positions where only the lowest-paying jobs were within their reach. The drive toward a more stable life situation has been described by other researchers as well (Baumann, 1994; Montgomery, 1994). However, current policy and program responses to homelessness tend to focus on short-term solutions (e.g., emergency shelters), appear to do little to disrupt the cycle of homelessness, and in fact may just render women and children who are homeless less visible in the public eye (Weinreb & Buckner, 1993).

The notion of marginalization is relevant here. Marginalization means lack of integration (Galheigo, 2005) or pushing people to the periphery of society (Allahar, 1989), and women who are homeless seem to fit the definition of a marginalized population. The occupational concerns described in the current study suggest that women who are homeless wish to have the education, jobs and resources that would allow them to live the way others live and participate in the occupations that are typical. So what is keeping them marginalized?

Returning to the Canadian Model of Occupational Performance (CMOP), occupational therapists are reminded to attend to the person, the occupations people wish to engage in, and the impact of the environment in which the person is situated (Canadian Association of Occupational Therapists, 1997). When examining the occupational issues for homeless women with children, the striking factor is the impact of the institutional and social environments. Consider the participants' top five areas of occupational concern: finances, employment, education, transportation and housing. One might argue that the reason these women can't achieve these outcomes has something to do with spiritual, affective, cognitive and/or physical personal characteristics (the person component of CMOP), but this was not apparent at all from the study interviews.

Instead what stood out was the fact that the participants had limited educational backgrounds which made it difficult to obtain adequate employment that paid a living wage. More than half of the women had not completed high school, and none had completed college. It has been well-documented that it is almost impossible to raise a family on a job that pays minimum wage (National Coalition for the Homeless, 2003a). Lack of access to good salaries (note that the majority of women had an income of less than $800 per month) made it almost impossible to obtain stable housing. In fact, the disappearance of low-income housing has been documented as an important factor associated with the increase of homeless families (National Coalition for the Homeless, 2003b). In addition, inadequate financial resources made it difficult for the women to purchase reliable cars and instead they were forced to depend on a city public transportation system that is typically viewed by residents as inadequate. Institutional environmental factors including a wage structure that precludes financial independence, inadequate housing for the poor, and a deficient public transportation system appear to be key barriers precluding the women in this study from achieving their occupational goals.

An analysis of the social environment suggests that since inadequate financial resources made child care too expensive to afford, the women were unable to work unless they had social support to share the responsibility of caring for their children. This was not an option for women who were escaping relationships with partners or family members who were abusive. Thus, the social environment served as another barrier to development of the financial independence needed in order to address a variety of other occupational concerns.

This analysis suggests that environmental barriers are keeping the women in this study from engaging successfully in occupations in the areas of self-care, productivity and leisure. As described in the *International Classification of Functioning, Disability and Health* (World Health Organization, 2001), participation in the environment is the highest level of social inclusion, and to be barred from participation is beginning to be described by some occupational therapists as occupational injustice (Townsend & Wilcock, 2004). It is a serious charge to suggest that women with children who are homeless experience occupational injustice, but it is consistent with the understanding that they have become marginalized citizens who lack social inclusion, face institutional barriers, and are unable to participate in a full range of occupations that are available to others and typically encouraged as part of adulthood.

Implications for Occupational Therapy Practice

Townsend and Whiteford (2005) suggest a participatory occupational justice framework to use with populations who experience barriers to participation in everyday life. The framework consists of six non-linear, interrelated processes including:

- Analyzing occupational injustices (What qualitative and quantitative data exists concerning injustice?)
- Evaluating strengths, resources and challenges (What are client issues and strengths?)
- Negotiating a justice framework (What conflicting and congruent values and power issues need attention?)
- Negotiating program designs, outcomes and evaluations (What outcomes will be targeted and how will these be effected and measured?)
- Analyzing and coordinating resources (What resources are available and how will coordination be done?)
- Implementing and evaluating services (What services will have the greatest impact, how will they be carried out, and how will the effects be measured?)

These processes are all relevant to this small, descriptive study which suggests that women with children who are homeless *do experience occupational injustice.* That analysis moves us to consider also the other processes in the framework. An *evaluation of the participants' strengths, resources and challenges* would require more in-depth discussion of the occupational issues and concerns raised by the COPM. This evaluation needs to be client-centered and empowering (Canadian Association of Occupational Therapists, 1991). That is, the occupational therapist and client would need to collaborate to develop a joint understanding of the woman's personal and environmental strengths, resources, and areas of difficulty.

Negotiating an occupational justice framework is equivalent to choosing a theoretical approach. The occupational therapist and women will need to clarify how they see the problem . . . what approaches have been tried, what avenues appear to have utility? This allows everyone to work together as they come to agreement about the underlying source of the occupational issues.

Other components of the occupational justice framework in this situation involve *choosing a program design, clarifying what resources are available and how best to use them,* and *actually implementing and evaluating services*. The key issue here is to determine the best way to actually address the occupational issues and concerns. Deciding when to target personal changes and when to target environmental changes will require careful thought. For example, if transportation is a problem, when is it appropriate for the occupational therapist to work with an individual on a plan to be able to borrow and eventually buy a car, and when is it appropriate to mobilize support and advocate with local government agencies for a more effective public transportation system? These are not easy questions, and they move occupational therapists from the more familiar territory of individual and small group-focused practice to the more unfamiliar terrain of political advocacy and activism.

In addition, it will also be important for occupational therapists to be constantly mindful of power relationships and the need to support the transfer of power from the occupational therapist to the person served (Urbanowski, 2005). Empowerment creates a momentum that takes persons beyond solving the current problem, and facilitates their development as an active occupational agent in creating a meaningful, satisfying life. Some of the women in this study told us that nobody had ever asked them to tell their story before. The simple fact of sitting down in a private place, and asking them to talk about their daily occupational routines and issues helped them to become visible, and helped them to begin to think about how they wanted life to be.

This descriptive study exploring the occupational concerns of 27 women who are homeless with children raises many more questions than it answers. How do we identify when we are working with populations that experience occupational injustice? What models of analysis are most effective to use? How do we as occupational therapists respond to instances of occupational injustice at the individual and/or system level? What is the proper role of occupational therapy and what are the needed skills and tools to allow effective professional responses? These are important questions that occupational therapists will need to explore more deeply in order to assure interventions that facilitate full occupational participation and social justice for marginalized populations such as homeless women and families.

REFERENCES

Allahar, A. (1989). *Sociology and the periphery: Theories and issues.* Toronto, CA: Garamond Press.

Banyard, V., & Graham-Bermann, S. (1995). Building an empowerment policy paradigm: Self-reported strengths of homeless mothers. *American Journal of Orthopsychiatry, 65,* 479-491.

Bassuk, E.L., Buckner, J.C., Weinreb, L.F., Browne, A., Bassuk, S.S., Dawson, R. et al. (1997). Homelessness in female-headed families: Childhood and adult risk and protective factors. *American Journal of Public Health, 87,* 241-247.

Bassuk, E.L., Weinreb, L.F., Buckner, J.C., Browne, A., Solomon, A., & Bassuk, S.S. (1996). The characteristics and needs of sheltered homeless and low-income housed mothers. *Journal of American Medical Association, 276,* 640-646.

Baumann, S.L. (1994). No place of their own: An exploratory study. *Nursing Science Quarterly, 7,* 162-169.

Burt, M., Aron, L.Y., Lee, E., & Valente, J. (2001). *Helping America's homeless: Emergency shelter or affordable housing.* Washington, DC: The Urban Institute Press.

Canadian Association of Occupational Therapists (1991). *Occupational therapy guidelines for client-centered practice.* Toronto, ON: CAOT Publications.

Canadian Association of Occupational Therapists (1997). *Enabling occupation: An occupational therapy perspective.* Ottawa, ON: CAOT Publications.

Chan, C., & Lee, T. (1997). Validity of the Canadian Occupational Therapy Measure. *Occupational Therapy International, 4,* 229-247.

Davis, J., & Kutter, C.J. (1998). Independent living skills and posttraumatic stress disorder in women who are homeless: Implications for future practice. *American Journal of Occupational Therapy, 52,* 39-44.

Drake, M. (1992). Level I fieldwork in a daycare for homeless children. *Occupational Therapy in Health Care, 8,* 215-224.

Finlayson, M., Baker, M., Rodman, L., & Herzberg, G. (2002). The process and outcomes of a multimethod needs assessment at a homeless shelter. *American Journal of Occupational Therapy, 56,* 313-321.

Galheigo, S.M. (2005). Occupational therapy and the social field. In F. Kronenberg, S. Simo Algado, & N. Pollard (Eds.), *Occupational therapy without borders: Learning from the spirit of survivors* (pp. 87-98). Edinburgh: Elsevier.

Herzberg, G., & Finlayson, M. (2001). Development of occupational therapy in a homeless shelter. *Occupational Therapy in Health Care, 13,* 133-147.

Heubner, J., & Tryssenaar, J. (1996). Development of an occupational therapy practice perspective in a homeless shelter: A fieldwork experience. *Canadian Journal of Occupational Therapy, 63,* 24-32.

Kavanagh, J., & Fares, J. (1995). Using the model of human occupation with homeless mentally ill clients. *British Journal of Occupational Therapy, 58,* 419-422.

Kroening, C. (2002). *Women who are homeless with children: Time use, space use, and childcare assistance.* Unpublished master's thesis, University of New Mexico, Albuquerque, NM.

Law, M., Baptiste, S., Carswell, A., McColl, M.A., Polatajko, H., & Pollock, N. (1998). *Canadian Occupational Performance Measure, third edition.* Ottawa, Canada: CAOT Publications ACE.

McColl, M.A., Paterson, M., Davies, D., Doubt, L., & Law, M. (1999). Validity and community utility of the Canadian Occupational Performance Measure. *Canadian Journal of Occupational Therapy, 67,* 22-30.

Mitchell, H., & Jones, J. (1997). Homelessness: A review of the social policy background and the role of occupational therapy. *British Journal of Occupational Therapy, 60,* 315-319.

Montgomery, C. (1994). Swimming upstream: The strengths of women who survive homelessness. *Advanced Nursing Science, 16*(3), 34-45.

National Coalition for the Homeless (2003a). *People need livable incomes* (NCH Fact Sheet). Retrieved August 14, 2005 from the World Wide Web: http://www.national homeless.org/facts/income.html

National Coalition for the Homeless (2003b). *People need affordable housing* (NCH Fact Sheet). Retrieved August 14, 2005 from the World Wide Web: http://www.nationalhomeless.org/facts/housing.html

Nunez, R., & Fox, C. (1999). A snapshot of family homelessness across America. *Political Science Quarterly, 114,* 289-307.

Nyamathi, A., & Flaskerud, J. (1992). A community-based inventory of current concerns of impoverished homeless and drug-addicted minority women. *Research in Nursing & Health, 15,* 121-129.

Ripat, J., Etcheverry, E., Cooper, J., & Tate, R. (2001). A comparison of the Canadian Occupational Therapy Measure and the Health Assessment Questionnaire. *Canadian Journal of Occupational Therapy, 68,* 247-253.

Rossi, P.H. (1994). Troubling families: Family homelessness in America. *American Behavioral Scientist, 37,* 342-395.

Roth, L., & Fox, E.R. (1990). Children of homeless families: Health status and access to health care. *Journal of Community Health, 15,* 275-284.

Schultz-Krohn, W. (2004). The meaning of family routines in a homeless shelter. *American Journal of Occupational Therapy, 58,* 531-542.

Toomey, M., Nicholson, D., & Carswell, A. (1995). The clinical utility of the Canadian Occupational Performance Measure. *Canadian Journal of Occupational Therapy, 62,* 242-249.

Townsend, E., & Whiteford, G. (2005). A participatory occupational therapy justice framework: Population-based processes of practice. In F. Kronenberg, S. Simo Algado, & N. Pollard (Eds.), *Occupational therapy without borders: Learning from the spirit of survivors* (pp. 110-126). Edinburgh: Elsevier.

Townsend, E., & Wilcock, A. (2004). Occupational justice. In C.H. Christiansen & E. A. Townsend (Eds.), *Introduction to occupation: The art and science of living* (pp. 243-273). Upper Saddle River, NJ: Prentice Hall.

Tryssenaar, J., Jones, E.J., & Lee, D. (1999). Occupational performance needs of a shelter population. *Canadian Journal of Occupational Therapy, 66,* 188-96.

Urbanowski, R. (2005). Transcending practice borders through perspective transformation. In F. Kronenberg, S. Simo Algado, & N. Pollard (Eds.), *Occupational therapy without borders: Learning from the spirit of survivors* (pp. 87-98). Edinburgh: Elsevier.

U.S. Conference of Mayors (2001). *A status report on hunger and homelessness in America's cities: A 27-city survey.* Washington, DC. Retrieved from http://usmayors.org

Weinreb, L., & Buckner, J.C. (1993). Homeless families: Program responses and public policies. *American Journal of Orthopsychiatry, 63,* 400-409.

World Health Organization (2001). *The international classification of functioning, disability and health.* Geneva: World Health Organization.

doi:10.1300/J003v20n03_04

Describing the Phenomenon of Homelessness Through the Theory of Occupational Adaptation

Jennifer A. Johnson, PhD, OTR/L

SUMMARY. The purpose of this study was to illustrate the value of the theory of Occupational Adaptation (Schkade & Schultz, 1992; Schultz & Schkade, 1992) in describing the phenomenon of homelessness. Case studies portray the experience of four individuals residing in a homeless shelter. Utilizing Occupational Adaptation to guide the assessment and intervention process, the results suggest that this theory may be useful in describing the individuals' internal adaptation process necessary to live independent and productive lives. doi:10.1300/J003v20n03_05 *[Article copies available for a fee from The Haworth Document Delivery Service: 1-800-HAWORTH. E-mail address: <docdelivery@haworthpress.com> Website: <http://www.HaworthPress.com> © 2006 by The Haworth Press, Inc. All rights reserved.]*

KEYWORDS. Occupational Adaptation, homelessness, occupational therapy, adaptation

---

Jennifer A. Johnson is affiliated with the University of Central Arkansas, Department of Occupational Therapy, 201 Donaghey Avenue, Doyne Health Science Center, Suite 300, Conway, AR 72035 (E-mail: jennifer@uca.edu).

The author is grateful to Dr. Sally Schultz, Dr. Janette Schkade, and Dr. Rob Kennedy for their expertise and guidance during the research project. The author appreciates the individuals who participated in the study.

[Haworth co-indexing entry note]: "Describing the Phenomenon of Homelessness Through the Theory of Occupational Adaptation." Johnson, Jennifer A. Co-published simultaneously in *Occupational Therapy in Health Care* (The Haworth Press, Inc.) Vol. 20, No. 3/4, 2006, pp. 63-80; and: *Homelessness in America: Perspectives, Characterizations, and Considerations for Occupational Therapy* (ed: Kathleen Swenson Miller, Georgiana L. Herzberg, and Sharon A. Ray) The Haworth Press, Inc., 2006, pp. 63-80. Single or multiple copies of this article are available for a fee from The Haworth Document Delivery Service [1-800-HAWORTH, 9:00 a.m. - 5:00 p.m. (EST). E-mail address: docdelivery@haworthpress.com].

Available online at http://othc.haworthpress.com
© 2006 by The Haworth Press, Inc. All rights reserved.
doi:10.1300/J003v20n03_05

Recognized as a significant social problem in the United States, homelessness affects about 3.5 million people (Burt, Aron, & Lee, 2001). The majority of the homeless population range in age between 25 to 45 years of age. Forty-eight percent of the homeless have never been married and 24% have been divorced.

Homeless individuals experience a number of complex problems because homelessness is not merely a housing issue. The unremitting stresses related to homelessness and the basic needs for survival are constant tests for these individuals (Buckner, Bassuk, & Zima, 1993; Jencks, 1994). Noteworthy problems associated with homelessness include physical or sexual abuse, lack of social support, and poor self-esteem (DiBlasio & Belcher, 1993; Herman, Susser, Struening, & Link, 1997; Johnson, Freels, Parson, & Vangest, 1997; Kingree, Stephens, Braithwaite, & Griffin, 1999). Homelessness "inevitably disrupts the sense of identity and feelings of self-worth and self-efficacy" (Buckner, Bassuk, & Zima, 1993, p. 385).

Mental illness and addiction disorders or substance abuse are significant problems found associated with homelessness (Johnson et al., 1997; North, Pollio, Smith, & Spitznagel, 1998; Wuerker, 1997). Although the literature has indicated a relationship between addiction disorders, mental illness, and homelessness, there is a debate regarding which of these factors causes the other. Substance abuse and psychiatric disorders may be both causative of and precipitated by homelessness as suggested in the literature (North et al., 1998; Wuerker, 1997). Johnson et al. (1997) indicated that homeless individuals might abuse drugs and alcohol in an attempt to self-medicate psychiatric health problems. At the same time, research on the timing that homelessness occurs in relation to the onset of mental illness or substance abuse appears to indicate that homelessness generally occurs after one of the other variables has appeared (Johnson et al., 1997; North et al., 1998). This implies that psychiatric disorders and substance abuse may cause or at least create vulnerability to homelessness.

The primary services that exist for the homeless individuals are shelters and soup kitchens. These facilities respond to basic emergency needs for food and protection from the elements (National Coalition of Homeless, 1998). Services may include assistance with food and clothing, health-care referrals, case management, transportation needs, social work, and counseling for substance abuse, mental illness, and abusive relationships. Also offered are legal services, job training and placement, religious services, child care, education, housing referrals, and financial assistance. While programming exists to assist individuals who are homeless, homelessness has not seemed to diminish (Burt, Aron, & Lee, 2001). It is the opinion of this researcher that the development of day-to-day living skills appears to be a highly significant but an overlooked necessity for successful use of all the services provided.

In view of the increasing number of homeless individuals, the complex problems they experience, and the unique role of occupational therapy in community settings, this researcher acknowledges the potential benefits of occupational therapy. Moreover, while scholars in occupational therapy have investigated the factors contributing to homelessness, the meaning of the experience, and plausible intervention strategies (Finlayson, Baker, Rodman, & Herzberg, 2002; Miller, Bunch-Harrison, Brumbaugh, Kutty, & FitzGerald, 2005; Schultz-Krohn, 2004), this researcher asserts that describing the phenomenon of homelessness would be valuable. More specifically, this researcher is proposing that the theory of Occupational Adaptation (Schkade & Schultz, 1992; Schultz & Schkade, 1992) can be useful in understanding homelessness from an occupational therapy point of view.

THE THEORY OF OCCUPATIONAL ADAPTATION

Occupational Adaptation (OA) is a theory that describes a "normal" process of internal adaptation that occurs in human beings (Schkade & Schultz, 1992; Schultz & Schkade, 1992). In addition, the theory provides the occupational therapy practitioner with a framework that guides assessment and intervention. It assists the occupational therapist in facilitating an individual's ability to make adaptations to engage in activities that are personally meaningful (Schkade & Schultz, 1992; Schultz & Schkade, 1992). Through using an individually selected role and goal to guide intervention, the function of the individual's internal adaptation process is enhanced. The occupational therapist evaluates the individual's ability to carry out the activities within that chosen role and determines what is helping or hindering the individual from accomplishing his or her goal. An intervention plan is then developed to enhance the individual's capabilities.

Occupational Adaptation emphasizes the interaction between the person and the environment (Schkade & Schultz, 1992). In the theory, the person consists of three systems (sensorimotor, cognitive, and psychosocial) that interact with the occupational environment (physical, social, and cultural). Occupational Adaptation posits that as the person and the environment come together, there is a press for mastery that results in an occupational challenge or goal. As the individual responds to the challenges that arise, a process known as the adaptive response generation subprocess occurs in the person. This subprocess is the anticipatory portion of the adaptation process and the point at which occupational therapy intervention can play a pivotal role (Schkade & McClung, 2001).

> This subprocess is characterized by two components: the adaptive response mechanism and the adaptation gestalt. The adaptive response mechanism is the energy that drives the process (adaptation energy), the patterns of responding to challenges that have developed with time and experience (adaptive response modes), and the particular behavior types or classes that the person uses in an attempt to respond adaptively (adaptive response behaviors). (Schkade & McClung, 2001, p. 33)

Occupational Adaptation asserts that there are two levels of adaptation energy (primary and secondary) in which individuals operate. Primary adaptation energy is active when the individual is highly focused (e.g., trying to think of a person's name) on the task, and secondary adaptation energy is active when the individual is able to be more sophisticated and creative (e.g., remembers the person's name while watching television that evening).

> Adaptive response modes are classified as existing adaptive response modes (those already in our repertoire), modified adaptive response modes (those in which we make changes in an existing mode), and new adaptive response modes (those that come about because our existing or modified modes are not working for a particular need). (Schkade & McClung, 2001, p. 37)

Finally, the adaptive response behaviors are classified as primitive or hyperstable (all person systems are frozen and no adaptive behavior is occurring), transitional or hypermobile (high activity level and random behaviors in all person systems), and mature (goal-directed behaviors leading to adaptive responses) (Schkade & McClung, 2001).

Once the adaptation response generation subprocess has resulted in an occupational response, an evaluation occurs in both the person and the environment. This subprocess is known as the "adaptive response evaluation subprocess." It is at this time when the individual evaluates how they feel they performed in terms of "relative mastery." "Relative mastery is the extent to which the person experiences the occupational response as efficient (time and energy), effective (production of the desired result), and satisfying to self and society" (Schkade & Schultz, 1992, p. 835). In addition, this is the time when the person can observe whether the response reflects changes in the occupational adaptation process. According to OA, adaptation occurs when: (a) self-initiated adaptations are made; (b) relative mastery is enhanced; and (c) generalization occurs with new activities. This evaluation process leads to learning, which is an internal process that occurs, and influences performance.

Occupational Adaptation posits that "in order to improve occupational functioning, the intervention must be directly related to the patient's occupations of daily living or a particular occupational challenge" (Schultz & Schkade, 1992, p. 918). Therefore, the role of the occupational therapist that follows OA is to "function as the agent of the patient's occupational environment" and allow the patient to interact meaningfully with his/her environment (Schultz & Schkade, 1992, p. 918). The goal of intervention is to affect the person's internal adaptation capabilities.

METHOD

Researchers, using the theory of Occupational Adaptation, met with four individuals who were homeless. The participants were residents drawn from a homeless shelter located in a southern community with a population of approximately 50,000 residents. This 20-bed shelter, designed to assist with transitional housing, provides basic services as well as casework management. The length of stay at the shelter ranges from two weeks to two years; the average length of time a resident resides at the shelter is five months. The subjects were, by necessity, a sample of convenience that met the criteria for inclusion (ages 20 to 65, not actively psychotic or suicidal, or under the influence of drugs or alcohol).

Procedure

The researcher and an assistant who was an entry-level Masters student in occupational therapy met with each participant individually to discuss the purpose and procedures of the study. It should be noted that the assistant had received instruction through course work regarding OA. In addition, the assistant met with the researcher four times for instruction regarding OA and the research procedures. Additionally, the researcher and the assistant met once a week to discuss the progress of the research and address any questions.

Ten individuals who met the inclusion criteria agreed to participate in the study. However, only four of the participants completed the entire study; the remaining participants left the shelter after only one or two meetings. After obtaining informed consent, each participant worked with the researchers approximately two times a week, an hour at a time, for eight weeks. The researcher utilized OA in the evaluation and intervention process (Schkade & Schultz, 1992; Schultz & Schkade, 1992). The therapeutic climate of the sessions was collaborative in nature. The sessions consisted of the client and the occupational therapist identifying an occupational challenge(s) or goal, the therapist evaluating the individual and the environment that facilitated or inhibited the individual's ability to meet that challenge, and collaborative development of strategies in order to meet the occupational challenge. The occupational therapist served as a consultant or facilitator, a role that permitted the client to function as his or her own agent of change. The occupational therapist suggested activities, provided guidance, and offered feedback based on the client's actions and responses.

Following each session, the researcher documented the participant's actions, responses, and outcomes relevant to the OA process. In addition, the researcher recorded observations and interpretations of the participant's adaptive process. The case studies described the use of OA in terms of conceptualizing the phenomenon of homelessness. Review of the documentation yielded insights into the participant's experience. The components of the OA process, as described in the theory that consistently emerged from the case studies, were utilized in order to describe the homeless experience.

RESULTS

For the sake of discussion, one case study will be used as an exemplar in describing the use of OA. The other three case studies will be described in brief detail in Tables 1, 2, and 3.

Case Study

Peggy is a 57-year-old woman who had been residing at the shelter for four months prior to the study. She reported that she could no longer support herself and this was the second time she had been homeless. Peggy looked her age with no apparent physical or sensory problems. She did not

TABLE 1. Case Study Shauna

	Shauna
Person	24-year-old female; Independent with mobility although abnormal posture; Facial features disfigured; Impaired speech. *Cognitive functioning*–follows directions, answers questions, performs job duties, but demonstrated impaired judgment skills; *Psychosocial* functioning is impaired as evidenced by social relationships and the handling of these relationships and reported lack of social support
Occupational Environment(s)	Prior to residing at the shelter, participant lived in another state constantly moving from city to city; Moved away from home because her "mother did not want her to live there"; Stated that her mother had numerous boyfriends moving in and out; Job history included approximately 20 jobs primarily in food service and janitorial work
Occupational Roles	Unable to define any *occupational roles*; Through conversations in later sessions, resident described herself as a friend
Occupational Challenge(s)	Move back to Michigan
Adaptive Response Generation Subprocess	*Energy level–primary*–focused on getting "home" to Michigan–every activity focused on getting back to Michigan, but all involved her in a passive role; *Adaptive Response Mode–pre-existing* as evidenced by the numerous jobs she has had and lost due to poor performance. Majority of relationships were mutually beneficial; Constantly moving away from people or situations that do not seem to work out; *Adaptive Response Behavior–transitional (hypermobile)* as evidenced by her "hopping" from one task to another. Difficulty staying on task
Adaptation	Coping, but little evidence of adaptation. Did seek out homeless shelter, but this is a common solution for her when things are not going well and she needs a place to stay; The only *self-initiation* she demonstrated was seeking out previous activities in order to obtain money; *Relative mastery* fluctuates from high to low on any given day; No evidence of *generalization*

Italicized words denote concepts from the Theory of Occupational Adaptation

have a vehicle so she walked anywhere she needed to go. Peggy's cognitive functioning appeared to be normal. She was able to describe her life history and insights into her current situation. Since she had been at the shelter for four months, the director had assigned her some administrative duties. Psychosocially, Peggy demonstrated some difficulty. She ap-

TABLE 2. Case Study Brian

	Brian
Person	39-year-old male; *Sensorimotor* functioning was within normal limits; *Cognitive* functioning appeared intact. He reported difficulty with concentration; Stated that although he graduated from high school, he had difficulty with most subjects; *Psychosocial* functioning appeared impaired as evidenced by the participant's reported choice of people he develops relationships with and how he handles the situations; Minimal contact with family
Occupational Environment(s)	Prior to residing at the shelter, he lived in Colorado with his girlfriend. He stated living in many places, but sister lived in city where homeless shelter is located; Reported numerous jobs–all requiring physical labor. During time of intervention, participant worked for a moving company
Occupational Roles	He identified himself as a worker, brother, and self-maintainer
Occupational Challenge(s)	Initially, just wanted to get off the street; Following several sessions, participant reported wanting to save money to buy a car (although his license had been suspended for DUI's), get his own place, find a girlfriend, go to some type of school or get vocational training, and keep a job
Adaptive Response Generation Subprocess	*Energy levels*–evidence of both *primary* and *secondary*. Sometimes very focused (*primary*) on getting out of the shelter and at times *secondary* as evidenced by seeking out additional employment opportunities in order to learn a new trade; *Adaptive Response Mode*–prior to intervention there was evidence of *pre-existing mode* of behavior (substance abuse, losing job, back to substance abuse); By end of intervention, there was evidence of *modified* and *new modes of behaviors* as evidenced by maintaining job, staying away from drugs and previous social network, focused on "turning life around"
Adaptation	Initially, coping skills (as opposed to adaptation) to "survive" as evidenced by numerous times he had been to the shelter; End of intervention it appeared that signs of adaptation were occurring; *Self-initiation*–observed by seeking out additional learning opportunities; *Relative mastery*–initially very low "me against the world," but by end of intervention signs of improvement noted–identifying goals and feeling good about maintaining present job; *Generalization*–as evidenced by seeing success at maintaining job, now seeking out additional job opportunities

Italicized words denote concepts from the Theory of Occupational Adaptation

TABLE 3. Case Study Matt

	Matt
Person	25-year-old male; *Sensorimotor functioning* was intact. *Cognitive* and *psychosocial* functioning–documented bipolar personality disorder and borderline personality disorder; Participant demonstrated lack of judgment; Demonstrates impulsively; Currently receiving treatment for drug and alcohol abuse; Minimal contact with family although his father, brother, and sister live in the same city; Social contacts include those individuals with whom he engages in drugs and alcohol
Occupational Environment(s)	He was referred to the shelter by a day treatment program that "treated mental illness and substance abuse problems"; He was "kicked out" because he had broken some of the rules (taking drugs). The homeless shelter agreed to take him for a limited time since he had nowhere else to go. Prior to the shelter he lived in an apartment (low income) where he made several "friends who could get him drugs."
Occupational Roles	He spoke of roles that he previously had such as boyfriend, son, and brother. He reported that he would like to regain the roles, but was not observed to be active in any of them during time of study
Occupational Challenge(s)	Move and be married within the next 5 years; "Get out of institutions and get on the right medications"
Adaptive Response Generation Subprocess	*Energy level–primary* as evidenced by "I am afraid I cannot break set"; Stated that there were "too many steps to deal with"; *Adaptive response mode–pre-existing*–although thinking about making some changes, not active in doing it; Gets a job and then loses it again because of drug and alcohol abuse–ends up in institution or shelter; *Adaptive Response Behavior–primitive (hyperstable)* as evidenced by approach to goals (he could not express how to approach obtaining a goal)
Adaptation	No evidence of adaptation noted; No evidence of self-initiation of activities; Relative mastery remained low; No evidence of generalization

Italicized words denote concepts from the Theory of Occupational Adaptation

peared to lack the confidence in her ability to "do any better than I am right now." She lacked family and any social support other than what she was receiving through the shelter. She had adult children, but did not stay in touch with them. She had been married twice; both times ended in divorce "because both of them had drinking problems."

Occupational Environments

Peggy did not discuss her previous living situations: "it is too difficult for me to think about how I had to live." However, prior to this homeless episode she lived in a small house (in the same city as the shelter) with a friend. (She stated that she no longer had contact with this friend.) Peggy stated that she had to move because she could no longer afford the rent and utilities. At the time of the initial interviews, Peggy worked in a fast food restaurant "cooking fries." She stated that she had worked there for almost two years on a part-time basis. She stated that "fast food is really all I know." Peggy reported that she did not work when she was married and did not have any "formal training in any other type of work."

Occupational Roles

Peggy rarely discussed any other role than that of a worker. Anytime she was asked to describe the events of the day, she discussed activities related to work. She discussed the activities related to her employment and the "chores required around the shelter." She reported that she attended different churches on Sunday (a volunteer of the shelter would take her), but that she did not "belong to any one church." Although she reported having children, she did not discuss them until the fifth session. She stated that she never saw them. She did not report having any friends. Peggy stated that she did not "have anything in common with the kids" she worked with at the fast food restaurant.

Occupational Challenge

Peggy stated that she wanted to "live on my own." However, initially she did not have a detailed plan of how to obtain this goal. "I guess I will live here until I get enough money to live on my own." She also stated that she would like to join a church and "be active in it."

Adaptive Response Generation Subprocess

Peggy seemed to be going through the "motions" without a clear idea of what to do next. She appeared to be operating in primary energy because she focused on the fact that her life situation was always going to be the same. Peggy seemed satisfied or complacent since initially she was not able to identify the need to obtain more income than she was receiving in order to afford the expenses required to live independently.

She was going to keep the part-time job she had until she saved "enough money to move out."

Peggy appeared to operate primarily in a preexisting mode of behavior. For example, every time she was divorced she became homeless and moved into a shelter. Both of the men that she married had reported problems with alcohol. She "endures" each difficult situation with "this is how it is supposed to be, so why try to change it." She remained in the fast food business because "it is all I know" and does not think about attempting a different type of employment that might allow her to earn more income. When asked to identify her strengths regarding work she only stated that she was "dependable." "I have only missed two days of work in the last year and that was because I could not walk in the ice."

Peggy primarily operated in a primitive type of behavior. She is hyperstable in her way of thinking and behaving. For example, she was unable to identify any other options for employment. "I haven't thought of any other place to work." Peggy appeared "stuck" when asked to identify any other means for her to live independently. She only stated that "they (the shelter) have gotten me on the list for low-income housing, but they say that there is a three-year waiting list." She seemed satisfied with moving into a homeless shelter when "the money runs out." She was just waiting to save enough money to move out and then when she was no longer able to afford it she would move back into the shelter. . . "as long as I don't break any rules, I can come back and they (the shelter) would help me."

Evidence of Adaptation

It appeared that Peggy was coping with her life situation as opposed to making the necessary internal adaptations needed to live independently and productively. Coping "implies the use of personal resources and competencies to resolve stress and create new ways of dealing with problem situations" (Christiansen, 1991, p. 71). Adaptation, on the other hand, is a normative process that occurs continually over the lifespan of the individual. It is "a change in function that promotes survival and self-actualization" (AOTA, 1979, p. 785). Peggy seeks assistance when in need, but only uses the services provided to "correct" temporarily the problems. For example, she lives in the shelter just long enough for them (the shelter) to help her save money, obtain governmental assistance, and find housing. The shelter assists her with food, clothing, and furnishing of the housing whenever she seeks assistance. "Last time I left, they gave me some clothes, a television, and a pantry full of food to help me get started . . . and several times I needed help paying my utilities and they helped me." The researcher did not observe any change in Peggy's behavior as she responded to daily challenges; she only responded when encouraged to do something (i.e., filling out other job applications after it was suggested to her). This notion refers back to her primitive adaptive response behavior and existing mode of behavior. In addition, she did not engage in assessing her mastery or adaptation in order to make the necessary changes so that she might succeed.

There was little evidence of self-initiation in terms of Peggy identifying and pursuing an activity that would allow her to live independently. The majority of activities that Peggy engaged in were those initiated by an individual assisting her. When Peggy described her relative mastery related to the roles and activities in which she spent time, she stated that she was "fairly satisfied with how things are going." She stated that "if I had a place to live things would be better, but things are not bad here." "I would not mind working somewhere else, but at least I know what I am doing (at her present job)." There did not appear to be any evidence that Peggy was generalizing any knowledge or skills learned from life experiences or activities.

The information presented in Tables 1, 2, and 3 demonstrates the use of OA in identifying and describing the factors affecting the individuals who were homeless in this study. The tables give an overview of the homeless phenomenon based on the experiences and circumstances of the participants.

DISCUSSION

The results of this study illustrate the value of the theory of Occupational Adaptation in understanding homelessness. Occupational Adaptation provides worthy information and assistance that the traditional methods of evaluation (skill-based) with people who are homeless seem to lack. Occupational Adaptation views the person holistically by evaluating the sensorimotor, cognitive, and psychosocial aspects of the individual. An individual may lack the ability to live a productive life because of a problem in one of these areas. For example, Shauna had difficulty with speech because of her disfigured facial features. Her speech interfered with personal relationships, job opportunities, and self-esteem. Matt's cognitive subsystem was significantly impaired resulting in poor judgment and unpredictable actions. All of the participants demonstrated problems with psychosocial functioning whether it is a lack of social support or difficulty with personal relationships. Peggy was unable to name one person who she could ask for assistance in her time of need. Only after several meetings did she report having any children. The person system appears to be a logical, albeit complicated, area that should be addressed. However, it is highly overlooked by traditional methods of evaluation and treatment for people who are homeless. Another important area to address should be the environment in which the individual came from or currently performs their day-to-day activities. All of the participants were able to describe environments or components of those environments that inhibited productive living. For example, one of Matt's environments was his apartment (before he was evicted). The social and cultural environment of that apartment complex made it relatively easy for him to obtain drugs. Although he was in a treatment program to help him with his addiction, his "apartment environment" facilitated the opposite effect. Shauna's home environment was such that she felt she was not wanted because her mother had so many "boyfriends" moving in and out. Peggy's work environment in the fast food restaurant affected her ability to develop meaningful friendships because she was much older than the typical worker. The standard intervention plans do not appear to address the significant impact the environment has on the homeless individual. Additionally, this researcher could not find any evidence of an intervention program addressing the roles of the individual who is homeless and the effect their roles (or the lack of roles) have on them individually, their environment, or their ability to live an independent and productive life. Roles allow individuals to participate in society and satisfy human needs (Heard, 1977). For the most part, the participants in this study had few roles in which they were an active participant at the time of their homeless episode. Adults who live productive and satisfying lives engage in many roles such as parent, spouse, worker, student, friend, and volunteer. Dysfunctional role performance can lead to poor life satisfaction, lack of motivation, decrease feelings of self-esteem, and can produce social, psychological, and behavioral problems (Dickerson & Oakley, 1995; Versluys, 1980). Given what is known about the relationship between participation in roles and the ability to participate successfully in society, this is an area that requires further exploration with the homeless population.

The theory of Occupational Adaptation allows the occupational therapist to go beyond typical evaluation or intervention programs in that it addresses the person's ability to adapt internally. Living an independent and productive life depends on the ability to adapt. Adaptation allows individuals to meet the demands of the environment, cope with the problems of everyday living, and fulfill age-specific roles (Breines, 1986; Fidler &

Fidler, 1978). Adaptation is an accumulative process in which past experiences shape the future. It allows the individual to appraise new situations through looking at former ways of doing things and finding the best match or developing new ways to perform (Spencer, Davidson, & White, 1996).

Occupational Adaptation examines the process of adaptation by evaluating how the person goes about day-to-day activities and the challenges that arise. It is from this evaluation process that the individual and the occupational therapist can see why problems may arise. For example, in Peggy's case study, she exhibited a primitive (hyperstable) behavior in her thinking and acting as it related to changing jobs in order to increase her income. She stated that she had not thought about getting a job that provided more hours and increased pay. Shauna, on the other hand, was operating in a transitional (hypermobile) behavior that inhibited her from focusing on the important tasks. She seemed focused on whatever challenge arose that day and focused so intently (primary energy) on that challenge that she "forgot" what she was supposed to do. For example, Shauna wanted to use the phone to contact a man she met the day before, and at the shelter you must use a pay phone (she did not have any money). On the same day, a volunteer from the shelter was going to take her to several places of employment to fill out applications. Instead of obtaining the applications, she asked each of these places if she could use their phone. Although this may seem to be a trivial example, this was a common way for Shauna to react and behave. Matt's life story provides the reader with an example of his difficulty in self-initiating or generalizing positive things he learned as a boy growing up in a relatively stable environment and in the numerous "treatment programs." He is able to communicate the facilitators and consequences of drug and alcohol abuse and ways to prevent the use, but has been unsuccessful in overcoming the addiction. He stated that he knew that moving into that apartment would not be good "because many of his friends" lived there.

Occupational Adaptation can be invaluable to the occupational therapist working with a homeless individual. Although it may sound cliché, OA encourages the occupational therapist to look at the "whole person" and the environments in which they perform their daily activities. Evaluating the person systems allows the therapist to determine what basic factors may be preventing the individual from being able to perform successfully. For example, it was important to know that although Shauna graduated from high school, she participated in special education courses that assisted her throughout her academic career. Shauna may not have the intellectual capabilities necessary to hold certain types of jobs. Therefore, intervention in this area would focus on the process that Shauna would undertake in determining her capabilities that match her vocational interests and abilities.

The theory of OA posits that the occupational environment is as important as the client's physical or mental condition (Schultz & Schkade, 1992). Evaluating the environmental systems permits the occupational therapist to see what factors or situations may inhibit a person from living independently. For example, it was important to know that the apartment where Matt may be moving back to has people residing there with drug problems of their own. Matt lived in that apartment because of the close proximity to the day treatment center and relatively inexpensive rent. Intervention would focus on assisting Matt in realizing the problems with living in this environment and guiding him through a process that would encourage him to look at other plausible alternatives to housing.

Determining the roles (along with the responsibilities and expectations of these roles) in which these individuals actively participate is a significant piece of information that will allow the occupational therapist to understand how they spend their time and what or who is important to them. The lack of role participation among these participants tells the occupational therapist that they may not be spending their time wisely or productively. It also may alert the therapist that the individual may lack the motivation to participate in roles, lacks social support, or lacks the ability to function in a particular role. Intervention through consultation, guidance, instruction, or meaningful activities would focus on addressing the factors inhibiting successful role performance.

One of the most important aspects that seem to be missing from typical intervention programs is assessment and intervention based on what the client views as important and meaningful. It is important to know the challenges and goals of the individual. The theory of OA posits that in order for intervention to be effective (promote adaptation), the treatment program must be directly related to activities that are important and meaningful to the client (Schultz & Schkade, 1992). Therefore, by determining the client's goals and centering intervention on those goals, treatment will be more successful. For example, since one of Brian's goals was to "get his own place," intervention could focus on all that is required in obtaining a place of residence (saving money, determining cost of living, determining location, loan applications, etc.). This process of "getting his own place" will require him to develop competencies that will be useful in other situations in the future.

The evaluation process in the theory of OA (adaptive response generation subprocess) allows the client and the occupational therapist to identify modes and patterns of behavior. This component of OA assisted this researcher and the participants in determining and understanding why they (participants) were homeless and responded the way they did to certain situations. For example, Peggy applied for a job through a temporary employment agency (standard procedure at the homeless shelter). She was then asked to participate in an interview; however, she did not get the job. When asked if she could find out why she did not get the job or if this agency had any other jobs available, she stated that she "just figured there was no reason to. . . ." This researcher observed this typical response on a weekly basis. In order to change this behavior and allow Peggy to become her own "change agent" the occupational therapist should initially have a greater role in the treatment activities, but as therapy progresses, allowing Peggy's role to become greater. Identifying what is important to Peggy and utilizing the competencies gained from participation in those activities will serve to assist her in using those abilities in obtaining employment. In addition, it is important to note that Peggy rarely evaluated her performance. Without this evaluation process, change is not likely to occur. Therefore, the occupational therapist must assist Peggy in understanding the need for this self-evaluation. In addition, the occupational therapist represents part of the environment. Helping Peggy understand the expectations (society expects you to contribute) placed on her by the environment could be an important first step.

CONCLUSION

The needs of people who are homeless are great because homelessness is much more than not having a place to live. The literature and the case studies represented in this paper demonstrate the numerous difficulties and problems that exist with the homeless. Not only do these individuals struggle with obtaining the basic necessities such as food, clothing, and shelter; they may experience problems associated with drug and alcohol abuse, physical abuse, mental illness, diminished feelings of self-worth, and lack of control. It is evident that the homeless individuals represented in these case studies have many problems that affect all areas of their lives.

The theory of Occupational Adaptation enables the occupational therapist to understand the phenomenon of homelessness in order to create a successful intervention plan. It allows the occupational therapist to address all areas of the person, the environment, and their interaction (person/environment) in order to determine the area or areas that are inhibiting the normal process of adaptation.

REFERENCES

American Occupational Therapy Association (1979). Statement of philosophy. *American Journal of Occupational Therapy, 33*, 781-813.

Breines, E. (1986). *Origins and adaptations: A philosophy of practice.* Lebanon, NJ: Geri-Rehab, Inc.

Buckner, J. C., Bassuk, E. L., & Zima, M. D. (1993). Mental health issues affecting homeless women: Implications for intervention. *American Journal of Orthopsychiatry, 63*(3), 385-397.

Burt, M., Aron, L.Y., & Lee, E. (2001). *Helping America's homeless: Emergency shelter or affordable housing?* Washington, DC: Urban Institute Press.

Christiansen, C. (1991). Performance deficits as sources of stress: Coping theory and occupational therapy. In C. Christiansen & C. Baum (Eds.), *Occupational therapy: Overcoming human performance deficits* (pp. 69-96). Thorofare, NJ: Slack.

DiBlasio, F. A., & Belcher, J. R. (1993). Social work outreach to homeless people and the need to address issues of self-esteem. *Health and Social Work, 18*(4), 281-287.

Dickerson, A. E., & Oakley, F. (1995). Comparing the roles of community-living persons and patient populations. *American Journal of Occupational Therapy, 49*(3), 221-228.

Fidler, G. S., & Fidler, J. W. (1978). Doing and becoming: Purposeful action and self-actualization. *American Journal of Occupational Therapy, 32*(5), 305-310.

Finlayson, M., Baker, M., Rodman, L., & Herzberg, G. (2002). The process and outcomes of a multimethod needs assessment at a homeless shelter. *American Journal of Occupational Therapy, 56*(3), 313-321.

Heard, C. (1977). Occupational role acquisition: A perspective on the chronically disabled. *American Journal of Occupational Therapy, 31,* 243-247.

Herman, D. B., Susser, E. S., Struening, E. L., & Link, B. L. (1997). Adverse childhood experiences: Are they risk factors for adult homeless? *American Journal of Public Health, 87*(2), 249- 255.

Jencks, C. (1994). *The homeless.* Cambridge, MA: Harvard University Press.

Johnson, T. P., Freels, S. A., Parson, J. A., & Vangest, J. B. (1997). Substance abuse and homelessness: Social selection or social adaptation? *Addiction, 92*(4), 437- 445.

Kingree, J. B., Stephens, T., Braithwaite, R., & Griffin, J. (1999). Predictors of homelessness among participants in a substance abuse treatment program. *American Journal of Orthopsychiatry, 69*(2), 261-266.

Miller, K., Bunch-Harrison, S., Brumbaugh, B., Kutty, R., & FitzGerald, K. (2005). The meaning of computers to a group of men who are homeless. *American Journal of Occupational Therapy, 59*(2), 191-197.

North, C. S., Pollio, D. E., Smith, E. M., & Spitznagel, E. L. (1998). Correlates of early onset and chronicity of homelessness in a large urban homeless population. *The Journal of Nervous and Mental Disease, 186*(7), 393- 400.

Schkade, J., & McClung, M. (2001). *Occupational adaptation in practice.* Thorofare, NJ: Slack.

Schkade, J., & Schultz, S. (1992). Occupational adaptation: Toward a holistic approach for contemporary practice, part 1. *American Journal of Occupational Therapy, 46*(9), 829-837.

Schultz, S., & Schkade, J. (1992). Occupational adaptation: Toward a holistic approach for contemporary practice, part 2. *American Journal of Occupational Therapy, 46*(10), 917-925.

Schultz-Krohn, W. (2004). The meaning of family routines in a homeless shelter. *American Journal of Occupational Therapy, 58*(5), 531-542.

Spencer, J., Davidson, H., & White, V. (1996). Continuity and change: Past experience as adaptive repertoire in occupational adaptation. *American Journal of Occupational Therapy, 50*(7), 526-534.

Versluys, H. (1980). The remediation of role disorders through focused group work. *American Journal of Occupational Therapy, 35*(9), 609-614.

Wuerker, A. K. (1997). Factors in the transition to homelessness in the chronically mentally ill. *Journal of Social Distress and the Homeless, 6*(3), 251-260.

doi:10.1300/J003v20n03_05

Mother-Toddler Interactions During Child-Focused Activity in Transitional Housing

Sharon A. Ray, ScD, OTR/L

SUMMARY. This report describes the videotaped interactions of five mother-toddler dyads living in transitional housing. This study was designed to specifically examine the interactions as a function of routine in different types of child-focused activity. The interactions were described using the Parent-Toddler Coding System and Rating Scales of Dyadic Interaction (Ray & Tickle-Degnen, 2004). The focus was to examine the socio-emotional and task-supporting interactions that relate to the child's engagement in child-focused activity. Interactions were examined during free play, block play, slide play, and while having a snack. Positive moderate associations were noted between maternal and child socio-emotional dimensions of interactions in all activity conditions. The associations between maternal socio-emotional and task-related dimensions of interactions with child task-related dimensions of interaction were small in a positive direction, with higher associations noted in more familiar tasks such as during slide play or while having a snack. These preliminary findings suggest that familiarity

Sharon A. Ray, ScD, OTR/L, is Assistant Professor of Occupational Therapy at Tufts University, Medford, MA.

Address correspondence to: (sharon.ray@tufts.edu).

[Haworth co-indexing entry note]: "Mother-Toddler Interactions During Child-Focused Activity in Transitional Housing." Ray, Sharon A. Co-published simultaneously in *Occupational Therapy in Health Care* (The Haworth Press, Inc.) Vol. 20, No. 3/4, 2006, pp. 81-97; and: *Homelessness in America: Perspectives, Characterizations, and Considerations for Occupational Therapy* (ed: Kathleen Swenson Miller, Georgiana L. Herzberg, and Sharon A. Ray) The Haworth Press, Inc., 2006, pp. 81-97. Single or multiple copies of this article are available for a fee from The Haworth Document Delivery Service [1-800-HAWORTH, 9:00 a.m. - 5:00 p.m. (EST). E-mail address: docdelivery@haworthpress.com].

Available online at http://othc.haworthpress.com
© 2006 by The Haworth Press, Inc. All rights reserved.
doi:10.1300/J003v20n03_06

with routines should be considered when examining the interactions that support child activity in families living in transitional housing for the homeless. doi:10.1300/J003v20n03_06 *[Article copies available for a fee from The Haworth Document Delivery Service: 1-800-HAWORTH. E-mail address: <docdelivery@haworthpress.com> Website: <http://www.HaworthPress.com>* *© 2006 by The Haworth Press, Inc. All rights reserved.]*

KEYWORDS. Mother-child interaction, homelessness, child activity, context

INTRODUCTION

Increasing numbers of families in poverty are residing in shelters for the homeless (Children's Defense Fund, 2004) and the young children living in these families are at risk for behavioral, developmental, and health concerns (Anooshian, 2005; Bassuk, 1990; Bassuk et al., 1997; Bassuk & Rosenberg, 1990; O'Neil-Pirozzi, 2003; Youngblade & Mulville, 1998). There has been some evidence that delays may be primarily due to the condition of poverty (Coll, Buckner, Brooks, Weinrub, & Bassuk, 1998). Occupational therapists provide services to families at risk through early intervention programs. One of the mechanisms that they use to support child development is the mother-child relationship. However, the research has been done with families living in stable housing (Kinderman, 1993; Rogoff, 1990; Rollins, 2003; Zaslow et al., 2006). It is not known whether the same mechanisms to support child action are effective when the child and caregiver are confronted with the social and physical environment that characterizes life in transitional homes. This exploratory study reports an analysis of the interactions between mothers and toddlers residing in transitional housing. The purpose of this study is to examine the mother-toddler interactions that occur during child-focused activities. The interactions were explored during different types of play activities and while having a snack.

Importance of Parent-Child Interaction

Qualities of the parent-child relationship have been shown to be related to the developmental status of the child (Belsky, Goode, & Most, 1980; Rollins, 2003; Rogoff, 1990). Interactions between the child and caregiver have been shown to be a primary mechanism through which the child acquires language, play, and self-care skills (Murray & Hornbaker, 1997; Vibbert & Bornstein, 1989). Although this topic has been much studied in families living in regular housing, there has been no research that examined these mechanisms in homeless families or families living in transitional housing.

Developmentalists view the relationship between the toddler in the second year of life and the caregiver as essential in supporting development of the child's affective and didactic or task-related skills (Rogoff, 1990; Stern, 1995). According to Vygotsky (1978), these skills do not develop independently but within the context of the child's culture, and the adults in the child's life provide important support for the child's skill acquisition. The adults provide meaning to the child's activity and use the interactions to help the child learn about family roles and routines (Stern, 1995). Activity occurs within a social context and within a physical context that includes the materials that are the object of the action as well as the physical environment. The parent uses the physical setting and materials of the activity as the context that helps to shape the child's participation (Rogoff, 1990).

Description of Parent-Toddler Interaction

The child and caregiver create an interaction history that supports the child's action and language. The interaction history is used for the establishment of attitudes, expectation of behavior, and understanding of roles during shared activity (Sroufe & Fleeson, 1986). The child learns the expectation for how to participate in activities including the manner of task accomplishment and role as a participant in the activity such as a leader, follower, or cooperative participant (Ninio & Bruner, 1976; Stern, 1995). The child's participation in activities is shaped through joint problem-solving and collaborative play.

The caregiver provides a continuum of support, from verbally and physically controlling the child's actions, to encouraging independent participation (Frodi, Bridges, & Grolnick, 1985). In studies of toddlers entering the second year (Kinderman, 1993; Vibbert & Bornstein, 1989), mothers were found to adjust their behaviors to their perception of child competence during motor and self-care tasks. The mothers tended to ignore the child's attempts at independent action and would complete the tasks for the child when the child was not perceived as developmentally ready to participate. When the child was perceived as more competent, competence was facilitated by ignoring immature attempts and substituting more mature behaviors (Kinderman, 1993). Heckhausen (1987) found that caregivers use the child's attempts to accomplish a task as a marker of competence rather than age. This approach necessitates the caregiver's sensitivity to the child's action.

Children's participation in activities is shaped by their relationship with the caregiver. Sroufe and Fleeson (1986) found that toddlers explore more when the caregiver is in the child's visual field and is watching, than when the caregiver's attention is directed elsewhere. Belsky and colleagues (1980) found that the child's exploratory competence was related to maternal interventions to support play. Physical support included actions such as demonstration or repositioning of materials. These actions have stronger associations with child action than verbal support such as directing or instructing the child. Directive behavior has been found to be associated with child persistence but not competence or positive affect (Frodi et al., 1985).

The physical setting and materials are also instrumental in shaping the interactions that support the child's participation. In a study of toddler play, the caregivers were found to adjust their task-related speech more to the play materials rather than to the actions of the child. More varied and affective speech was associated with symbolic play toys while more informational styles were used with toys such as blocks or shape sorters (O'Brien & Nagle, 1986). Wachs (1987) found that the availability of toys was related to the amount of object play. The caregiver's demonstration of object play and nonverbal responses to object play were related to social object mastery. The child was able to enlist the caregiver's involvement through the use of objects and such actions as offering to share. Thus, in addition to the interaction shaping the child's participation in activity, the physical setting and materials also shape the mother-child relationship during child-focused activity.

Description of Parent-Toddler Interaction in Shelters

Rogoff (1990) discussed the role of location as an important factor in setting the context for interactions. The nature of transitional housing is to provide temporary shelter. In the Massachusetts shelters that provided subjects for this study, the typical length of stay is six to nine months. For families, moving to a new setting requires the development of new routines that are adapted to the new environment. The adjustment may include the use of shared spaces for activities such as meals, play, and other leisure time activities. Families may have a history of using shared spaces before entering the shelter, however, the temporary nature of the shelter requires a family to renegotiate their routines as new residents come to the shelter. In addition to adjusting to the new physical setting, families need to adjust to new routines for everyday tasks. A study of families in a shelter in Atlanta (Boxill & Beatty, 1990) found that mothers may have limited opportunities to develop relationships with their children in private, due to shared space for meals and living spaces. Mothers also reported a loss of traditional parental roles such as meal planning and preparation and determining the family schedule or activities.

The purpose of this study was to describe the interactions between mothers and toddlers living in transitional housing during different types of activity, in particular, the relationships between caregiver socio-emotional and task-related action and child action. The interactions were examined during typical family routines such as engaging in a meal or snack and in leisure time activities of the families' choosing, and also while engaging in novel routines using props provided by the researcher. The interactions were videotaped within each family's shelter residence in order to examine the interactions as they might be influenced by this environmental context. Interaction trends were described by the type of interactions that occurred using the Parent-Toddler Coding System and the Rating Scales of Dyadic Interaction (Ray & Tickle-Degnen, 2004).

METHOD

Participants

Five mother-toddler dyads living in transitional housing in the greater Boston area completed the study. The dyads had been in the shelter for one to five months at the time of their participation in the study. The demographic information for these five dyads is reported in Table 1. The toddlers had no reported medical or neurological concerns. None of the toddlers had siblings.

Measures

The videotaped interactions were analyzed using the Parent-Toddler Coding System (PTCS) and the Rating Scales of Dyadic Interaction (RSDI) (Ray & Tickle-Degnen, 2004). Each tool describes both the task-related and socio-emotional behaviors of the mother and child. The PTCS was used to code the presence or absence of behaviors of the mother and child during interactions. An example of task-related behavior for mother or child is imitation, and of socio-emotional behavior is hugging.

TABLE 1. Characteristics of the Subject Pairs

Mother			Child					
Subject Pair	Age in years	Educational Degree	Age in Months	Gender	Ethnicity	Bayley II Scores Mental	Motor	In group childcare
1	20	In GED program	14	Female	Biracial[a] White Hispanic	106	80	No
2	17	In GED program	17	Male	Biracial[a] White Black	98	94	Yes
3	19	In GED program	18	Female	White	91	107	Yes
4	28	High school	12	Female	White	117	97	Yes
5	32	High school	14	Female	White	108	116	Yes

[a]For biracial children, the first ethnic category reflects the ethnicity of the mother.

The RSDI was used to describe subjective qualities of the interaction using the averaged ratings of 10 judges with experience working with young children and their families. An example of a maternal task-related RSDI quality is directiveness and a child quality is assistance-seeking. An example of a RSDI socio-emotional quality for the mother and child is playfulness. All items included in the study had interrater reliability greater than .90.

Procedure

Following informed consent, each toddler received a developmental assessment using the Bayley Scales (Bayley, 1993). Each mother participated in an interview to discover the history that led to living in transitional housing, her perspective of life in the residence, and her description of the relationship with her toddler. The mother-toddler dyad was videotaped during three 40-minute sessions in the subjects' residence within a two-week period. The schedule of the taping varied with each dyad in order to fit into their schedules. The videotaped sessions involved 10 minutes each of unstructured free play, play with two-inch blocks, play on a toddler-sized slide, and eating a typical snack or meal provided by the mother. During the free play segment the mothers were instructed to spend time with their child in their usual manner. The blocks and slide were provided by the investigator and the mothers were instructed to include these props in their interaction with no specific instruction given on how they should be included. These segments provided opportunities to observe comparable play situations across subjects. The snack segment provided an opportunity to examine the types of interactions that might occur during a meal.

Video clips were taken at 1, 3, 5, 7, and 9 minutes into each activity segment in order to obtain a sampling of behavior over time for each type of segment (free play, block play, slide play, and snack). Five 60-second clips were created for each of the four 4 10-minute activity segments for coding with the PTCS. Thirty-second clips were taken at the same intervals for judging using the RSDI.

Data Analysis

A principal components analysis was performed on the PTCS coded data for each type of activity. The parent items were analyzed separately from the child items. The factors were used to form the composite variables that were the unit for each analysis. Composites were formed so that the variables would reflect multiple dimensions of each attribute such as a positive socio-emotional variable reflecting both verbal and nonverbal socio-emotional behavior. The parent and child items were averaged to form task-related and socio-emotional composite variables (see Table 2). The parent task-related variables were Directs attention, Encourages participation, and Supports participation. The parent socio-emotional variable was labeled Expresses affection. The child task-related variables

TABLE 2. Description of the Items that Were Averaged to Form the Socio-Emotional and Task-Related Composite Variables from the Parent-Toddler Coding System (PTCS) and Rating Scales of Dyadic Interaction (RSDI) Using Principal Components Analyses

Averaged Variables	PTCS Composite Items	RSDI Composite Items
Socio-emotional	Expresses affection	Reflects affect
Task-related	Directs attention Encourages participation Supports participation	Structures Task Maintains attention
Child		
Socio-emotional	Demonstrates affection Displays emotion	Reflects affect
Task-related	Exerts independence Includes parent	Determines participation Initiates proximity

were Exerts independence and Includes parent, and the socio-emotional variables were Shows affection and Displays emotion.

A similar procedure was followed for the rated data of the RSDI. Principal components analyses were used to form the composite variables that were used for this study. The parent task-related variable was labeled Task organization and the socio-emotional variable was labeled Reflects positive affect. The task-related variable was Determines participation and the socio-emotional variables were Reflects affect and Initiates proximity (see Table 2).

Correlational matrices were formed to examine relations between the composite variables that described the interaction between child and parent in each of the four activity conditions (free play, block play, slide play, snack). The correlations for each subject pair were averaged by performing a *z* transformation in order to get an average correlation for each set of variables across subject pairs. The correlations were then averaged using *z* transformations to create the averaged correlations that included all of the correlations between mother and child (see Table 3).

The interactions were examined using the Structured Analysis of Social Behavior model (SASB) (Benjamin, 1987) for describing family interactions including verbal and nonverbal behaviors and the environmental context. The model can be used to describe the level of engagement occurring within the interaction using three types of interactions. Complementary interactions describe groups of behaviors that act as a function of each other such as when a child participates in a task to the mother's direction. Reciprocal interactions are when the behaviors of one of the pair elicit similar behaviors in the partner such as when each person

TABLE 3. Correlations Between Parent and Child Averaged Socio-Emotional and Task-Related Behavior by Type of Activity

Parent with Child	Activity			
	Play			
	Free	Block	Slide	Snack
Socio-emotional/Socio-emotional	**<u>.60</u>**	**.45**	**<u>.55</u>**	**.41**
Socio-emotional/Task-Related	.12	.05	**.30**	**.30**
Task-related/Task-Related	.25	.11	**.35**	**.32**
Task-Related/Socio-emotional	**.34**	**.34**	**.45**	.24

Note. $n = 15$ observations each of five subject pairs for each type of activity. The correlations are averaged across all subjects and all sessions. Parent and child task-related variables and socio-emotional variables are averaged separately. All correlations ≥ .30 are in bold print. All correlations of ≥ .50 are underlined.

expresses positive socio-emotional affect such as mutual smiling or touching. Strong positive associations between interaction variables describe high engagement that could be either reciprocal or complementary. Antithetical interactions are a type of disengagement and are defined as when the behavior observed is the opposite of the expected response such as a cry in response to a smile. In this study, antithetical interactions are shown by negative associations between interaction variables. Antithetical interactions might be typical of behaviors noted during child noncompliance or decreased maternal sensitivity. Interaction trends were also examined in terms of the type of interactions that occurred. The interactions were described as being socio-emotional or task-related using the Parent-Toddler Coding System and the Rating Scales of Dyadic Interaction (Ray & Tickle-Degnen, 2004).

RESULTS

Descriptions of the Socio-Emotional Dimensions of Interactions

According to Benjamin (1987), strong positive correlations between socio-emotional variables would suggest a level of high engagement. Strong negative correlations between maternal and child variables describe disrupted engagement. Table 3 shows that the socio-emotional dimensions of interactions between mother and child were moderate to strong in all activity conditions. There were strong positive average correlations across all activity conditions (average $r = .51$).

Description of the Task-Related Dimensions of Interactions

Table 3 shows that the average association between maternal socio-emotional and child task-related variables was small ($r = .20$). The average association between maternal and child task-related variables was also small ($r = .27$). The average association between maternal task-related variables with child socio-emotional variables was moderate ($r = .35$).

Description of the Interactions by Activity

Table 3 describes the relationship between parent and child socio-emotional variables for each type of activity. Moderate to strong positive associations were noted between the parent and child socio-emotional variables in all activity conditions, with the highest associations noted during free play ($r = .60$) and slide play ($r = .55$). The associations between maternal socio-emotional and task-related variables with child task-related variables were lower in the free play and block play conditions (averaged $r = .13$). The associations during slide play and snack were higher ($r = .30$).

There were small positive associations between the parent and child task-related items in the free ($r = .25$) and block play ($r = .11$) activity conditions and moderate positive associations in the slide play ($r = .35$) and snack ($r = .32$) activity conditions. The associations between maternal task-related variables and child socio-emotional variables were highest during the slide play condition ($r = .45$) and lowest during the snack condition ($r = .24$). The associations were similar in the free play and block play conditions ($r = .34$).

DISCUSSION

This preliminary study identified several interaction trends for families living in transitional housing. Strong engagement as defined by Benjamin (1987) occurred between socio-emotional behaviors of the mothers and toddlers in all activity conditions. Strong socio-emotional engagement involves interaction behaviors used to display positive affection such as hugging, smiling, or getting into a lap. These interaction behaviors are not dependent on a specific physical setting or the use of physical props or materials. Thus, if these socio-emotional interaction patterns were established prior to entering the shelter, they might be easier to continue because the behaviors require only the presence of each partner of the dyad. Socio-emotional engagement was lower when the activity condition demands required more task-supporting intervention by the parent as in the block play and snack conditions. Block play required intervention by the mother to give ideas for play and all of the toddlers were working on mastering self-feeding during snack, which required maternal support.

The associations between parent variables and child task-related variables showed a different pattern. Task-related engagement was lower than socio-emotional engagement in all activity conditions. This finding may suggest that the dyads did not have interaction routines as strongly established for child-supported activity. It might also suggest that during child-focused activity the child was exerting autonomy, a one-year-old developmental task, and was working on independent play rather than interaction with the mother.

Task-related engagement was sensitive to whether the activity condition involved established routines or whether the activity involved novelty. The highest task-related engagement, or the strongest associations of maternal behaviors with child task-related behaviors, occurred during snack and slide play. Both of these activity conditions were familiar to the mothers. During their interviews, all of the mothers stated that they were all responsible for feeding their children. Each of the subject pairs had established routines around the feeding episodes. Even if the meals were not in a consistent place or on a consistent schedule, the mother was always the primary person who fed or provided food for her child. The mothers reported that one of their primary concerns was the nourishment of their children. This is consistent with the finding of Wehler and associates (2004) who found that hunger was a primary concern in a study of families living in Massachusetts shelters. During snack times, the dyads engaged in interactions that involved both positive socio-emotional and task-related dimensions. All of the mothers reported having experience with slide play and each dyad showed moderate engagement during this activity condition.

Task-related engagement was low during free play and block play. Although the mothers expressed affection for their children during their interviews, they made statements suggesting that they did not know how to play with their children. One of the mothers stopped during the videotaping and said: "I don't know what to do." During the free play and block play videotaped segments, the dyads tended to approach each of these conditions as novel and thus did not appear to have established routines for play. In contrast, the subject pairs seemed to be able to establish routines for slide play. Although the toddlers did not have previous experience on the slide, it was an activity that was familiar to the mothers who quickly established a routine for play. The mothers shaped the play for their children initially but the dyads engaged in interactions that included both positive socio-emotional and task-related qualities.

The subject pairs in this sample had several challenges that are not typically seen in the population of housed families usually studied in research on mother-child interactions. The challenges were in the areas of physical environment, available materials, and social environment. All of the mothers reported that they were still adjusting to their life in the transitional housing. Four of the dyads did not have a consistent place for either play or feeding interactions and were still developing play and self-care routines at the time of the taping. An additional environmental factor was the presence of auditory and visual distractions inherent from living in shared quarters. Each of the dyads' videotaped sessions was interrupted by another person in the residence. In many of the tapes there were other residents' voices in the background. These features presented the additional challenge of screening out irrelevant stimuli while focusing on the targeted task.

Studies examining child skill acquisition have shown that children develop competence by building on established routines for participation in activity with significant adults. A factor in supporting child mastery is the provision of consistent materials for use as a prop in the interaction (Frodi et al., 1983; Ganea, 2005; Heckhausen, 1987; Rovee-Collier & Gulya, 2000). In order to support scaffolded learning, routines are developed and expanded with consistent materials used in child-focused activity. Four of the five dyads did not have their own toys and borrowed different toys from the community play room each session. The fifth pair had few toys. Mothers reported having to put their belongings in storage before entering the residences and toys were not considered a necessity. Different toys were used as props for each videotaped session for each dyad except for pair three, and no dyads beside pair three had established play routines. The mother of pair three had had previous experience with young children. Consistent interaction trends were noted during the snack segments. Most of the dyads had established feeding routines and all expressed concerns about their children having adequate nutrition. The consistent use of materials and routines during snack might explain the higher task-related engagement noted in snack when compared to play segments.

Similar to other research on parent-child interaction, the strongest reciprocal relationships were between the maternal and child socio-emotional variables. It was expected that maternal socio-emotional and child task behaviors would have stronger relationships than the associations between maternal and child task-related behaviors (Kinderman, 1993; Spangler, 1990; Vibbert & Bornstein, 1989). For example, both Vibbert and Bornstein (1989) and Wachs (1987) found the maternal socio-emotional behaviors to be the strongest predictor of both child play behavior and use of language. Other research findings have shown that directiveness, although a common tactic, was not an effective strategy in enticing a child to activity. Kuczynski and associates (1987) found that maternal directing behavior had strong associations with child noncompliance and direct defiance in children in the second year of life. One interpretation of the similar associations between maternal socio-emotional or task-related variables with child task-related variables is that the ability to establish a routine might be a more salient issue than the types of strategies used to establish those routines. The interaction associations were the same magnitude for both maternal socio-emotional and task-related dimensions of interactions with child task-related variables. The moderate associations between the maternal task-related variables and child socio-emotional variables might also suggest that the toddlers responded to the attention during child-focused activity except during snack where there was a clear expectation for the child to eat.

The results of this study show that it is possible to describe parent-child interaction trends in a population living in transitional housing using videotape methodology that is sensitive to the type of activity that the dyad engaged in. The results were consistent with other research in that it demonstrated positive socio-emotional interaction trends in all activity conditions. It was interesting that associations between maternal actions and child task-related actions appeared to be related to familiarity with routines in this exploratory research. Further study is needed to specifically test the hypothesis that familiarity with routines will impact the interactions during child-focused activities in this population. It would also be interesting to explore the mechanism through which an activity becomes familiar. During the present study the dyads quickly adapted to the use of the novel slide but a similar adjustment was not made to the use of the blocks supplied by the investigator. It would be interesting to explore the role of type of play, such as large motor play on the slide versus manipulative play as in the use of the blocks, in examining the mechanism of novelty and the establishment of play routines.

Consistent materials and activities may influence the interactions. During the free play segment of the session, the dyad was free to choose their activity. In this sample, much of the session was focused on play with manipulatives or other small toys. It would be interesting to investigate whether the interaction patterns observed were related to novelty in this population or with the type of activity, specifically the use of small toys. The involvement in small motor versus large motor play might explain why the interaction patterns during slide play were different than with either free or block play.

Further study is indicated using larger-sized samples. Of particular interest would be the effect of established routines when describing parent-child interaction in families living in shelters. A study of a sample with a shared common shelter residence or residence set-up is indicated to see if consistent interaction trends are present when the environment is more controlled. The relevant issues are the shelter routine, the control the mother has over schedules and routines, the use of private spaces, and the opportunity for consistent materials. Another important influence to consider is whether the child has a consistent day-care experience. The next step of this program study would be to explore the impact of this consistency on the child's developmental status.

The quality of play and interaction might have been impacted by the developmental range of the sample. There was a six month age range within the research sample. The toddlers were aged 12 to 18 months. Although the toddlers were all age-appropriate on the Bayley Scales of Infant Development (Bayley, 1993), they may have had different abilities in the use of language and play abilities. It might be useful to examine families with children closer in age.

Homelessness in families is a temporary condition and mothers in the sample did not define themselves by this condition. Longitudinal studies are indicated to examine whether the interaction patterns observed when living in transitional housing persisted when the families moved to stable housing. There was high engagement during snack; if other routines established during the play sequences carried over to stable housing situations, this would have implications for planning therapeutic interventions that focused upon the mother-child relationship in child development. It would be important to know whether the interaction patterns observed in the shelter were strongly reflective of the environmental content and would alter significantly in the context of a stable home. Although studies have examined the interaction patterns used by families living in poverty (Boxill & Beatty, 1990; Pianta & Egeland, 1990; Zaslow et al., 2006), it is not known whether the experience of homelessness has long-term effects on interaction patterns during child-focused activity.

IMPLICATIONS FOR OCCUPATIONAL THERAPY

This exploratory study adds to the knowledge base of occupational therapists who have an interest in families who live in transitional housing. There were trends in this study that suggest that the mechanisms for supporting child development and engagement in activity are consistent with studies of parent-child interaction in families living in more stable housing. Of particular interest were the reports of caring expressed by the mothers and the collaborative presence of strong socio-emotional engagement during all activity conditions. Consistent with the literature, positive socio-emotional interactions were more strongly associated with child-focused interaction than task-supporting interactions (Kinderman, 1993; Spangler, 1990; Vibbert & Bornstein, 1989; Wachs, 1987). In addition, familiarity of routine and materials appeared to be an important variable related to child activity engagement. The interaction patterns varied by the types of activities and materials used. Should these findings continue to be replicated in other studies, it would suggest that the use of familiar routines and materials as well as building on the socio-emotional interactions of families may be useful strategies for supporting mother-child interactions and child engagement in families living in transitional housing.

REFERENCES

Anooshian, L. J. (2005). Violence and aggression in the lives of homeless children: A review. *Aggression and Violent Behavior, 10*, 129-152.

Ayoun, C. (1998). Maternal responsiveness and search for hidden objects and contingency leaning by infants. *Early Development & Parenting, 7 (2)*, 61-72.

Bassuk, E. L. (1990). Who are the homeless families? Characteristics of sheltered mothers and children. *Community Mental Health Journal, 26*, 425-434.

Bassuk, E. L., Buckner, J. C., Weinreb, L. F., Browne, A., Bassuk, S. S., Dawson, R., & Perloff, J. N. (1997). Homelessness in female-headed families: Childhood and adult risk and protective factors. *American Journal of Public Health, 87*, 241-247.

Bassuk, E. L. & Rosenberg, L. (1990). Psychosocial characteristics of homeless children and children with homes. *Pediatrics, 85*, 257-261.

Bayley, N. (1993). *Bayley scales of infant development* (2nd ed.). San Antonio: Psychological Corporation.

Belsky, J., Goode, M. K., & Most, R. K. (1980). Maternal stimulation and infant exploratory competence: Cross sectional, correlational, and experimental analysis. *Child Development, 51*, 1152-1178.

Benjamin, L. S. (1987). An interpersonal approach. *Journal of Personality Disorders, 1*, 334-339.

Bornstein, M., Vibbert, M., Tal, J., & O'Donnell, K. (1992). Toddler language and play in the second year: Stability, covariation, and influences of parenting. *First Language, 12*, 323- 338.

Boxill, N. A. & Beatty, A. L. (1990). Mother/child interaction among homeless women and their children in a public shelter in Atlanta, Georgia. *Child and Youth Services, 14*, 49-64.

Children's Defense Fund (2004). *The state of America's children yearbook 2004*. Washington, DC: Children's Defense Fund.

Coll, C. G., Buckner, J. C., Brooks, M. G., Weinreb, L. F., & Bassuk, E. L. (1998). The developmental status and adaptive behavior of homeless and low-income housed infants and toddlers. *American Journal of Public Health, 88*, 1371-1374.

Frodi, A., Bridges, L., & Grolnick, W. (1985). Correlations of mastery-related behavior: A short term longitudinal study of infants in their second year. *Child Development, 56*, 1291-1298.

Ganea, P. A. (2005). Contextual factors affect absent reference comprehension in 14-month-olds. *Child Development, 76*, 989-998.

Heckhausen, J (1987). How do mothers know? Infants chronological age or performance as determinants of adaptation in maternal instruction. *Journal of Experimental Child Psychology, 43,* 212-226.

Kinderman, T.A. (1993). Fostering independence in mother-child interactions: Longitudinal changes in contingency patterns as children grow competent in developmental tasks. *International Journal of Behavioral Development, 16,* 513-535.

Kuczynsky, L., Kochanska, G., Radke-Yarrow, M., & Girnius-Brown, O. (1987) A developmental interpretation of young children's noncompliance. *Developmental Psychology, 23,* 799-806.

Murray, A. D. & Hornbaker, A. V. (1997). Maternal directive and facilitative interaction styles: Associations with language and cognitive development of low risk and high risk toddlers. *Development and Psychopathogy, 9,* 507-516.

Ninio, A. & Bruner, J. (1976). The achievement and antecedents of labeling. *Journal of Child Language, 5,* 1-15.

O'Brien, M. & Nagle, K. J. (1986). Parents' speech to toddlers: The effect of play context. *Journal of Child Language, 14,* 269-279.

O'Neil-Pirozzi, T. M. (2003). Language functioning of residents in family shelters. *American Journal of Speech-Language Pathology, 12,* 229-242.

Pianta, R. C. & Egeland, B. (1990). Life stress and parenting outcomes in a disadvantaged sample: Results of the mother-child interaction project. *Journal of Clinical Child Psychology, 19,* 329-336.

Ray, S. A. & Tickle-Degnen, L. (2004). The validity of a methodology to describe videotaped mother-toddler interactions. *Occupational Therapy Journal of Research, 24,* 123-133.

Rogoff, B. (1990). *Apprenticeship in thinking: Cognitive development in social context.* New York: Oxford Press.

Rollins, P. R. (2003). Caregivers' contingent comments to 9-month-old infants: Relationships with later language. *Applied Psycholinguistics, 24,* 221-234.

Rovee-Collier, C. & Gulya, M. (2000). Infant memory: Cues, contexts, categories, and lists. In D. L. Medin (Ed.), *The psychology of learning and motivation: Advances in research and theory* (pp. 1-46). San Diego: Academic Press.

Spangler, G. (1990). Mother, child, and situation correlates of toddler social competence. *Infant Mental Health Journal, 16,* 459-495.

Sroufe, L. A. & Fleeson, J. (1986). Attachment and the contribution of relationships. In W. W. Hartup & Z. Rubin (Eds.), *Relationships and development.* Hillsdale, NJ: Lawrence Erlbaum Associates.

Stern, D. (1995). *The motherhood constellation: A unified view of parent-infant psychotherapy.* New York: Basic Books.

The state of America's children yearbook 2004. Washington, DC: Children's Defense Fund.

Vibbert, M. & Bornstein, M. H. (1989). Specific associations between domains of mother-child interaction and toddler referential language and pretense play. *Infant Behavior and Development, 12,* 163-189.

Vygotsky, L. (1978). *Mind and society.* Cambridge, MA: Harvard University Press.

Wachs, T. D. (1987). Specificity of environmental action as manifest in environmental correlates of mastery motivation. *Developmental Psychology, 23,* 782-790.

Wehler, C., Weinreb, L. F., Huntington, N., Scott, R., Hosmer, D., Fletcher, K. et al. (2004). Risk and protective factors for adult and child hunger among low-income housed and homeless female-headed households. *American Journal of Public Health, 94,* 109-115.

Youngblade, L. M. & Mulville, B. A. (1998). Individual differences in homeless preschoolers' social behavior. *Journal of Applied Developmental Psychology, 19,* 593-614.

Zaslow, M. J., Weinfield, N. S., Gallagher, M., Hair, E. C., Ogawa, J. R., Egeland, B., Tabors, P. O., & Temple, J. M. (2006). Longitudinal prediction of child outcomes from different measures of parenting in a low income sample. *Developmental Psychology, 42*, 27-37.

doi:10.1300/J003v20n03_06

Homeless Youth: Causes, Consequences and the Role of Occupational Therapy

Ann M. Aviles, MS, OTR/L
Christine A. Helfrich, PhD, OTR/L

SUMMARY. This paper reviews the current literature on youth homelessness in the United States and the role of occupational therapy with this population. Youth homelessness is increasing with many youths becoming homeless due to a myriad of causes such as abusive situations in their homes and decreases in affordable housing. Definitions, causes, physical and mental health consequences and the impact of homelessness on youths' development into adult roles are discussed. The role of occupational therapy is described with a focus on useful assessments and intervention principles. Finally, a case study is presented to illustrate the use of these assessments and occupational therapy intervention with a female youth living in an emergency shelter. doi:10.1300/J003v20n03_07 *[Article copies available for a fee from The Haworth Document Delivery Service: 1-800-HAWORTH. E-mail address: <docdelivery@haworthpress.com> Website: <http://www.HaworthPress.com> © 2006 by The Haworth Press, Inc. All rights reserved.]*

Ann M. Aviles is Assistant Professor, Research Specialist in Health Sciences, Department of Psychiatry, University of Illinois at Chicago, 1747 W. Roosevelt Road, MC 747, RM 155, Chicago, IL 60608. Christine A. Helfrich is Assistant Professor, Department of Occupational Therapy, University of Illinois at Chicago, M/C 811, 1919 West Taylor Street, Chicago, IL 60612-7250.

This study was supported by grants from the Great Cities Faculty Seed Fund and the Campus Research Board at the University of Illinois at Chicago.

[Haworth co-indexing entry note]: "Homeless Youth: Causes, Consequences and the Role of Occupational Therapy." Aviles, Ann M., and Christine A. Helfrich. Co-published simultaneously in *Occupational Therapy in Health Care* (The Haworth Press, Inc.) Vol. 20, No. 3/4, 2006, pp. 99-114; and: *Homelessness in America: Perspectives, Characterizations, and Considerations for Occupational Therapy* (ed: Kathleen Swenson Miller, Georgiana L. Herzberg, and Sharon A. Ray) The Haworth Press, Inc., 2006, pp. 99-114. Single or multiple copies of this article are available for a fee from The Haworth Document Delivery Service [1-800-HAWORTH, 9:00 a.m. - 5:00 p.m. (EST). E-mail address: docdelivery@haworthpress.com].

Available online at http://othc.haworthpress.com
© 2006 by The Haworth Press, Inc. All rights reserved.
doi:10.1300/J003v20n03_07

KEYWORDS. Youth homelessness, youth development, life skills

INTRODUCTION

The number of homeless children has been increasing steadily, which can be explained, in part, by the shrinking labor market and decreases in affordable housing (www.nationalhomeless.org). Homelessness is associated with a myriad of problems for children and youth, one very important one being lack of life-skill development (Ensign, 2004). The aim of this paper is to review the current literature on youth homelessness and to describe occupational therapy's role in assessment and intervention with the homeless youth population. This paper will review the physical and mental health consequences faced by homeless youths, and the manner in which these factors impact their ability to complete daily life skills. A case study will be presented to illustrate occupational therapy's capacity to work with homeless youth on life-skill development.

BACKGROUND INFORMATION

The US Department of Justice estimated that in 1999, nearly 1.7 million youths had runaway/throwaway episodes that led to homelessness. Additionally, 25% of former foster care youths were homeless at least one night (Hammer, Finkelhor & Sedlak, 2002). These estimates may not truly reflect the number of homeless youths due to their transience and reluctance to seek out emergency shelter for fear of being returned to home, foster care, juvenile detention centers and psychiatric hospitalization (Greenblatt & Robertson, 1993; Kidd & Scrimenti, 2004). Despite the common belief that homeless youth are "out of control" youths who don't want to live by parental rules, this is far from the reality; instead, youths are often leaving situations of deprivation and abuse (Wrate & Blair, 1999). Research indicates that many homeless youth report abusive home environments (MacLean, Embry & Cauce, 1999). Additionally, youths experience family conflict over issues such as sexual activity, sexual orientation, pregnancy, school problems, and alcohol and drug use, resulting in additional youths who leave home and become homeless (Illinois Poverty Summit, 2004; Paradise & Cauce, 2002; Reeg, 2003). The complexity of factors contributing to homelessness among youths highlight some of the difficulties in studying this population. In examining the factors that contribute to homelessness among youth we must remember that there is a dynamic relationship that exists between adolescent development and the context(s) they inhabit. Adolescent development is best viewed within the context of family and social systems, as these are the primary systems they have contact with. Youths who are provided with support, guidance and a sense of connectedness to their world, in all contexts, will have better chances of reaching their full potential.

Homeless Youth Defined

Homeless youth are defined as individuals "not more than 21 years of age . . . for whom it is not possible to live in a safe environment with a relative and who has no other safe alternative living arrangement" (Reeg, 2003, p. 55). There are distinctions made within the category of homeless youth consisting of runaways (youths who have left home *voluntarily*), throwaways (youths told to leave home), street youth (youths living on the street) and systems youth (wards of the state) (Aviles & Helfrich, 2004). These categories of homeless youth are not mutually exclusive; rather, youths often move in and out of these categories dependent upon their particular situation. Additionally, the definition of "home" is not limited to traditional nuclear families, but also includes foster care, shelters, group homes and residential treatment facilities (Schaffner, 1998). It is also suggested that runaway youths leave home of their own will; however, it is often a response to familial conflict and/or abuse occurring in the home environment. Sixty to 80% of youths residing in homeless shelters and transitional living facilities report physical or sexual abuse by their parents or guardians prior to "running" away from home (Illinois Poverty Summit, 2004; Reeg, 2003).

Causes of Homelessness

Much of the literature on homeless youth focuses on youths who have runaway or those asked to leave home. However, the majority of homeless youth come from families that are suffering from instability (Chicago Coalition for the Homeless, 2001; Paradise & Cauce, 2002). More recently, emphasis has been placed on former foster care youths, estimating that 25-40% of former foster care youths become homeless (Illinois Poverty Summit, 2004). The parallels that exist between foster care youth and non-foster care youth point to the need to address the underlying issues that cause homelessness, specifically home environments plagued with abuse and neglect. Causes of homelessness among youth also consist of serious emotional disturbances, lack of affordable housing and an inability to secure affordable housing, lack of education and job skills, long-term family economic problems, violence in the home, absence of a parent and/or substance abuse by a parent (Chicago Coalition for the Homeless, 2001; Kidd & Scrimenti, 2004; www.endhomelessness.org). Additionally, youths embedded in families experiencing homelessness are often separated from them due to shelters that only allow young children to stay with their mothers, forcing older youths to care for themselves. It is important to note that pregnant and parenting teens, and youths who identify themselves as lesbian, gay, bisexual, transgendered or questioning (LGBTQ) are disproportionately represented among homeless youth (Chicago Coalition for the Homeless, 2001). The growing shortage of affordable housing and increases in poverty also contribute to homelessness (www.nationalhomeless.org).

Youths experiencing homelessness do so at different levels. Some youths may experience homelessness once or twice and may be reunited with their family, enter foster care or independent living. However, there are other youths who experience "chronic" homelessness, meaning that they continually experience homelessness. Youths who have chronic experiences with homelessness have a difficult time meeting basic needs such as acquiring food and shelter. Additionally, because they are on the street more, they are at greater risk for victimization, and physical and mental health problems (Lindsey, Kurtz, Jarvis, Williams & Nackerud, 2000).

Due to the varying causes and levels of homelessness experienced by youth it is important to note that homeless youth are not a homogenous group and therefore we must not make assumptions regarding their development of basic life skills. Youths' acquirement of life skills is dependent upon such factors as the age they became homeless, and the treatment they received (e.g., respect from adults, responsibilities given) while living in their homes (this includes "traditional" home environment, group home, foster home, etc.).

HEALTH CONSEQUENCES OF HOMELESSNESS

Physical Health

Homeless youth are a medically underserved population in the U.S. (Ensign, 2004). Homeless youth are at great risk for injuries, physical abuse, suicide, and homicide; approximately 5,000 per year die from assault, illness and suicide (Klein, Woods, Wilson, Prospero, Greene & Ringwalt, 2000). Some of the most common health problems identified by homeless youth consist of sexually transmitted diseases (STDs), Human Immunodeficiency Virus (HIV)/Acquired Immunodeficiency Syndrome (AIDS), pregnancy, dermatologic problems, malnutrition and injuries (Ensign & Gittelson, 1998). Despite youth being at greater risk for illness, they have significantly greater obstacles blocking their access to health-care than all other age groups (Klein et al., 2000). Youths who are able to access health-care consistently are often not provided with the opportunity to speak with their health-care provider privately to discuss sensitive issues such as pregnancy, HIV/AIDS and STDs (Ensign & Gittelson, 1998). Youths also lack the knowledge needed to access regular health-care, often relying on emergency rooms for their health-care needs. The emergency room is often their only access to care due to lack of insurance, confidentiality and embarrassment of their status as homeless youth (Klein et al., 2000; American Academy of Pediatrics [AAP], 1996). Despite youths' increased risk for injury and illness, they are less likely to seek out care due to their mistrust of adults (Klein et al., 2000)

Additionally, youths are viewed as minors by health-care providers; therefore, they often require parental consent, interfering with their ability to access health care. This is a clear indication of the misunderstanding health-care providers have of unaccompanied homeless youth seeking out health-care services. Youths who are not provided with the necessary services in emergency situations are often less likely to seek out preventative health care in non-emergency situations. As youths are attempting to secure basic needs such as food and shelter, health care becomes less of a priority (AAP, 1996). Many youths leave their communities when they become homeless and may not be familiar with the health services in a new community. Providers working with homeless youth should be aware of the health-care issues homeless youth face in addition to the barriers they encounter when attempting to seek out services in order to provide the appropriate resources youth need to access regular health care.

Mental Health

In addition to homeless youths' physical health needs, research also suggests homeless youth are more likely to demonstrate high rates of mental health problems (e.g., behavioral problems, depression, anxiety and self-harm) (Vostanis, Grattan, & Cumella, 1998). Mental health problems can be defined as behavioral and emotional difficulties causing concern or distress. The rates of mental health problems among homeless children/youth in the US are estimated to be 38% (Vostanis, 1999). Many of the risk factors that lead to homelessness have also been identified as risk factors for mental health problems such as violence in the home and mental illness among parents (Vostanis, 1999). Information regarding homeless youth indicates high rates of substance abuse, depression, mental illness and suicide attempts (Ensign & Gittelson, 1998; American Academy of Pediatrics, 1996). Unlike the perception of the seriousness of physical health, mental health is often not viewed as a "serious" problem. Many of the complex issues homeless youth face (e.g., abuse, involvement in the child welfare system) are related to underlying psychosocial factors (Vostanis et al., 1998). Furthermore, mental health problems have a negative stigma attached to them, making homeless youths even less likely to seek out services (Reid, 1999). Rather than seeking out mental health services, youths often self-medicate with street drugs (Reid, 1999).

A mental health problem common among homeless youth is post-traumatic stress disorder (PTSD) (Stewart, Steinman, Cauce, Cochran, Whitbeck & Hoyt, 2004). PTSD as defined by the Diagnostic and Statistical Manual of Mental Disorders (DSM-IV) (1994) is "the development of characteristic symptoms following exposure to an extreme traumatic stressor involving direct personal experience of an event that involves actual or threatened death or serious injury, or a threat to one's physical integrity" (p. 424). Many youths have experienced traumatic events in their homes that lead to their homeless situations, and are at-risk for victimization while homeless (Stewart et al., 2004), maintaining their vulnerability to PTSD and other mental health problems. PTSD symptoms such as avoidance, numbing and reexperiencing lead to self-injurious behaviors in homeless youth such as drug use, sexual promiscuity and gang involvement (Greenblatt & Robertson, 1993; Paradise & Cauce, 2002). Stewart et al. (2004) found that males are often victim to physical threats and assaults, and females to sexual exploitation and rape. The above study recognized the difficulty homeless youths face in securing basic needs such as food and shelter when they must also worry about being victimized.

Impact of Homelessness on Youth Development

The adolescent years are a critical time as youths are making their transition to adulthood. During this stage in life significant physical and emotional changes occur, making this a difficult time in life. An adolescent's access to resources that will support him/her in a successful transition to adulthood is essential to development. Adolescents require a stable foundation that consists of adults they can trust, and a safe, nurturing home environment. Unfortunately many adolescents have not had the privilege of being exposed to healthy environments, making adolescence an even more difficult stage of life.

The experiences homeless youth face exacerbate mental health problems such as aggression, depression, suicide, alcohol and drug use, and sexually transmitted diseases (Vostanis, Grattan, Cumella & Winchester, 1997). Mental health problems often lead to difficulties in social relationships and basic skills needed to negotiate various environments such as school and the workplace. Often youths rely on "survival" behaviors such as stealing, destruction of property, carrying a weapon for protection, panhandling, selling drugs or sex (survival sex), and forming gangs (Paradise & Cauce, 2002). Additionally, Greenblatt and Robertson (1993) recognize that homeless youths often surrender key relationships with adults, fail to develop work skills, rebel against formal institutions and abandon normative values after becoming homeless. Although these behaviors may be viewed as delinquent by authority figures (e.g., police, teachers, parents, etc.), oftentimes these behaviors are a sign of the strength of youths in their ability to survive their homeless experience.

The loss of "normative" experiences leads to poor or inappropriate development of basic life skills needed to successfully negotiate social institutions such as the workplace and school. Life skills are fundamental in supporting youth in becoming self-sufficient adults (Gourley, 2000). Life skills are often considered the domain of occupational therapy and lend themselves to an occupational therapy approach. Life skills consist of activities of daily living (bathing, dressing, grooming, eating) and instrumental activities of daily living (meal preparation, clothing care, cleaning, household maintenance, money management), and community skills (accessing transportation, time management, social interaction, community safety) (Okkema, 1993). When homeless youths experience a loss of traditional roles such as family member, student, worker, and friend they are often ill equipped to develop into healthy adults. Roth and Brooks-Gunn (2000) note "The numerous changes during adolescence appear to be overwhelming only for some adolescents–those with less optimal peer and family relationships, poorer coping skills . . . thus, circumstances from different environments–the family, peers, school–impact adolescents' preparation for, and success at navigating the transitions inherent in their development" (p. 4). Therefore, it is within the contexts of home and school that youths develop basic living skills, and for homeless youths this lack of contact with such environments often results in difficulties developing during adolescence and with their transition into adulthood. When youths are not afforded the opportunity to develop "traditional" adolescent roles, they instead develop "survival" roles (e.g., selling drugs). Forcing youths into adult roles without the appropriate preparation and support limits their ability to take on "normative" behaviors, which may lead to continued engagement of unhealthy behaviors as adults.

As discussed previously, the adversity homeless youth experience often leads to poor mental health, including their self-esteem. Self-esteem is defined as "the person's evaluation about self that expresses an attitude of approval or disapproval and indicates the extent to which the individual believes him or herself to be capable, significant, successful, and worthy" (Anderson & Olnhausen, 1999, p. 62). Youths who do not view themselves as "significant" or "worthy" due to their experiences of abuse and/or victimization may be less likely to care for themselves. Therefore, homeless youth may lack the "willingness to look at themselves and accept themselves as self-care agents and do not accept themselves as in need of or having the ability to perform particular self-care measures" (Anderson & Olnhausen, 1999, p. 63). Shelters provide housing, meals and referrals for various social and medical services; however, many times they do not teach youths the skills needed to access housing, food and other services on their own (Reid, 1999).

In order to better understand an individual's willingness and capability to perform the necessary life-skills needed to care for oneself, an investigation of multiple aspects of homeless youths' lives needs to be performed, including (but not limited to) how they became homeless, age they became homeless, physical and mental health and basic life skills, in order to provide services that will assist with their individual needs.

ASSESSMENT AND TREATMENT APPROACHES WITH HOMELESS YOUTH

Assessment

As discussed previously, youths' acquirement of life skills often depends on factors such as the age they became homeless, the treatment they received while living in their homes, as well as the length of time they have spent living in shelters and/or on the street. There are two assessments we have found useful with homeless youth, The Ansell-Casey Life Skill Assessment (ACLSA) and the Occupational Self-Assessment (OSA). Both of these assessments require input from the youths themselves and both acknowledge that youths have areas of strength that should be relied upon to address areas of concern.

The ACLSA is an evaluation of youth independent living skills. It assesses daily living tasks, housing and community resources, money management, self-care, social development (communication, relationships, community values), work and study habits (career planning, decision-making, study skills) (www.caseylifeskills.org/index.htm, accessed 1/15/05). The ACLSA has four versions which are age specific: ACLSA-I for ages 8-9 (37 questions), ACLSA-II for ages 10-12 (56 questions), ACLSA-III for ages 13-15 (81 questions), ACLSA-IV for ages 16-and-up (118 questions); also ACLSA short form for ages 11-18 (18 questions) (Casey Family Programs, 2005). Each version of the ACLSA recognizes youth within a developmental context, identifying the different skills attained as they negotiate adolescence. For example, at age 11 a youth would not be expected to have work skills, but one might expect those skills to be present by the age of 19; the different versions of the ACLSA account for such differentiation. The ACLSA demonstrates internal consistency, reliability, content validity, construct validity and test-retest reliability (Nollan, Horn, Downs & Pecora, 2002). Administration of the ACLSA takes approximately 30-45 minutes. The full-length assessments (ACLSA-I, ACLSA-II, ACLSA-III, ACLSA-IV) provide an overview of youth life-skills abilities. The ACLSA is useful for goal setting, program planning, and for measuring progress on life-skills acquisition. The short form assessment (ages 11-18) provides a brief summary of youth abilities. It is useful for evaluating programs and for getting a quick assessment of ability. There is also a Homeless Youth Assessment Supplement that assesses specific areas of concern to homeless youth.

The OSA assesses a person's occupational functioning and environment, measuring a youth's life-skills competence and the impact of the environment on his/her ability to adapt (Baron, Kielhofner, Goldhammer & Wolenski, 1999). This assessment allows youths to self-identify their areas of strength and weakness in regard to life skills, while simultaneously measuring how the environment(s) they function in support or inhibit their life-skill abilities. It also allows youths to identify areas of value, meaning that they categorize the skills that are most important to them in negotiating the different environments they encounter. When completing the OSA, youths rank how they are able to complete life skills through the following categories: "problem," "I do this all right," or "I do this well." Once they identify their ability to complete a task they rank how important it is to them, using a Likert format: "This is not so important to me," "This is important to me," or "This is extremely important to me." After completing the rankings for each item, the youth then identifies four items that s/he would like to change.

Both of these assessments rely on the youths' knowledge of their skills and abilities. Staff should have a well-established relationship with each individual so s/he will feel comfortable exploring and sharing skills that are not well-developed. The goal is for youths to recognize and understand that it is okay not to know and/or have specific skills. However, in order for them to be independent and negotiate multiple environments (e.g., workplace) acquisition of life skills is a necessity. Therefore, when assessing youths' skills we need to identify their existing strengths as well as identifying areas of need. Recognition of a youth's strengths can also help build a relationship between the youth and provider, as many homeless youths most often receive negative attention from adults. As providers we need to work with youths on seeing themselves as positive individuals capable of being self-sufficient adults. A study found that as youths begin to understand their experiences and themselves, they will gradually accept and value themselves in new ways, develop more self-confidence, take better care of themselves, take responsibility for their actions and trust potential helpers (Lindsey et al., 2000).

Treatment Principles

It is important for persons working with homeless youth to recognize and understand the barriers they encounter when attempting to access basic services. It is equally important to approach youths in a caring and respectful manner. Roth and Brooks-Gunn (2000) identify parental caring, connectedness and involvement with adolescents as of fundamental importance, being associated with better grades and educational expectations rather than delinquency and substance abuse. Therefore, youths who are not developing in supportive environments require programs that will provide a safe, "family like" environment, where caring adults will support and facilitate the development of life skills (Roth & Brooks-Gunn, 2000). Youths who are able to create strong relationships with adults (e.g., teachers, counselors) are less likely to engage in delinquent behaviors (Resnick, Bearman, Blum, Bauman, Harris, Jones, Tabor, Beuhring, Sieving, Shew, Ireland, Bearinger & Udry, 1997). Furthermore, creating trusting, caring relationships is necessary for a youth to feel comfortable and confident in asking adults for assistance in obtaining life-skill training. A study conducted by Kurtz et al. (2000) found that the quality most needed by homeless youths when interacting with providers was trust. The family context many homeless youths have fled from often prevents them from being able to trust others. Therefore, many youths find it difficult to confide in adults and ask for assistance. Many homeless youth have developed effective ways of keeping their distance from others in order to survive on the street. This may result in homeless adolescents struggling to adapt to a new environment, especially when leaving the streets and attempting to transition into a shelter or transitional housing facility (Levy, 1998). As providers we should be aware of the survival mechanisms youths have developed and be understanding of their reluctance to trust adults.

Providers need to recognize and emphasize youths' strengths and personal resources when working with them on their transition into adulthood, and hopefully out of homelessness. A study by Lindsey et al. (2000) identified two major criteria for homeless youths' successful navigation into adulthood: (1) personal strengths and resources; and (2) help received from others. This study highlights the importance of identifying the strengths homeless youth bring with them and the need to provide assistance in an effort to facilitate their ability to become successful adults. It is important to note that "success" should be defined by the youths themselves, rather than pressuring them to conform to societal norms. Although it is important for youths to recognize behaviors that interfere with their ability to be successful, youths that are able to come to such conclusions on their own often are motivated by their own desire to do well, rather than feeling obligated to do something based on the directions given by an adult. This is a hard balance to strike, as one needs to be helpful, supportive and firm but not overbearing or forceful. As many youths transition into adulthood they strive for autonomy and respect from adults, but they also continue to require advice and support from adults. This does not mean that a youth will follow the advice provided, and this may become very frustrating to providers working with homeless youth. As many of us progressed through adolescence we were given support and advice from parents, teachers, etc.; however, we often did not learn our lesson until we experienced the feeling of failure, disappointment, excitement, or happiness ourselves.

Providers must also understand the complexity of emotions youth are experiencing. Although youths are homeless due to family conflict, abuse, etc., many youths continue to have contact with their families. They may identify their families as the cause for becoming homeless, yet they continue to have relationships with them and often want to maintain these relationships despite the stress and strain it causes them. "Professionals who work with runaway and homeless youth need to recognize the importance of helping youth consider the possibility of reestablishing connections with family and friends who might be supportive and even engage in family counseling as appropriate to help resolve differences that keep youth and families apart" (Kurtz et al., 2000, p. 401).

The following case study illustrates the use of the assessments described previously and how occupational therapists can use the information obtained to plan an intervention.

Case Study

Angela is a 17-year-old female residing at an emergency youth shelter. Angela came to the shelter three years after being removed from her parent's home. Her parents were both addicted to drugs and often left her home alone to care for her younger siblings. She was removed from their home, due to neglect, at the age of 14 by child welfare services. Since that time Angela has lived with different relatives and in various shelters. She gave birth to a son at age 15. Shortly after his birth, she tried to commit suicide and was hospitalized for three months. Angela initially received psychiatric services and medication, but was unable to maintain these services when she became homeless. Her two-year-old son is developmentally delayed and received physical therapy services until they became homeless. She has been unable to manage health care for either of them due to their frequent mobility. Angela did not complete high school, but would like to obtain her GED and become employed. Angela expresses the importance of obtaining her education in order to "do something with my life." Angela has never been employed and would like to begin working, but does not have child care for her son. Angela has also stopped attending church, as she feels embarrassed because she does not have "appropriate" clothing to attend church.

Angela was able to identify areas of strength as well as areas of weakness on the Occupational Self Assessment (OSA). Angela's strengths include: (1) taking care of others for whom I am responsible (her son); (2) getting along with others; (3) expressing myself to others; and (4) taking care of myself. Areas Angela identified as problems include: (1) managing my basic needs (food, medicine); and (2) having a place where I can be productive (work, study, volunteer). Angela identified the following as areas she would like to improve: (1) working towards my goals; (2) handling my responsibilities; (3) identifying and solving problems; and (4) managing my finances. Information obtained from the ACLSA demonstrates Angela's lack of knowledge in daily living tasks, money management, and her work and study habits (career planning, decision-making, study skills). Her areas of strength include self-care and social development (communication, relationships, community values) and her ability to seek out housing and community resources.

One can see from these assessment results that each tool provided the occupational therapist with different, but complementary information about Angela. Angela demonstrated insight as she expressed to the occupational therapist that her current situation living in a homeless shelter and her unemployment status are limiting her ability to care for herself and her child. She is motivated to change her current situation but is not able to identify the steps needed to improve her situation.

The occupational therapist working with Angela was able to recognize her strengths. Angela is motivated, goal-oriented, able to self-evaluate, able to ask for assistance, and seeks out resources (sought out shelter and services within it). The shelter is providing her with temporary housing but she recognizes that she has a limited amount of time (120 days) until she will be responsible for herself and her child. Angela is receiving assistance with obtaining developmental services and child care for her son and mental health services for herself; however, she also expresses a need for assistance with identifying an approach that will allow her to work towards her goals, handle her responsibilities and successfully identify and solve problems she encounters in the process. While Angela identifies that she requires services to meet her basic needs, it is apparent that in order for her to sustain herself once she leaves the shelter she will need: (1) a provider that will work with her on identifying the actual steps needed to meet her goals; (2) brainstorm alternative situations; and (3) solutions that may arise as she works towards meeting her goals. In this process, it is vitally important that the provider emphasize Angela's strengths and use them as the vehicle for improvement.

The therapist and Angela engaged in activities such as role playing, to problem solve managing her basic needs (finances, working towards goals) in a safe environment with feedback from an adult. This provided her with opportunities to develop and practice life skills as well as the confidence to complete them successfully, contributing to the development of her self-confidence. Once Angela was able to work through problems via role playing, she and the therapist implemented these skills in the real world. Angela and the therapist visited the local bank, opened a savings account and worked on creating a budget; engaged in basic IADLs (laundry, simple meal prep); worked on filling out resumes, and engaged in mock interviews. Lastly Angela and the therapist sought out GED programs in the area. The therapist also met with Angela's case manager to discuss her mental health, resulting in a referral to the community mental health clinic in the shelter area. Angela's demonstration of life-skill development made her eligible for an independent living program for homeless teens with children where she will be able to continue to expand and hone her skills.

CONCLUSION

Homeless youth encounter many barriers limiting their ability to expand the life skills needed to engage in traditional roles of student, worker and family member. The reality of family conflict, lack of stable housing and victimization while living on the streets, negatively impact youths' physical and mental health. Youths' frequent lack of connection to caring and supportive adults hampers opportunities to cultivate strong, nurturing relationships that facilitate healthy adolescent development and successful transitions into adulthood. When youths become homeless, they may be unable to build and/or maintain routines and habits that afford them the opportunity to discover and expand life skills. As occupational therapists we are uniquely prepared to assess and identify a person's strengths and limitations. We are able to work with youth on creating and implementing an individual plan, fostering the skills needed to become a fully functional member of society. Collaborating with homeless youth in identifying life-skill needs and facilitating their development is a necessary component in occupational therapy treatment with the homeless youth population.

REFERENCES

American Academy of Pediatrics (1996). Health Needs of Homeless Children and Families. *Pediatrics, 98*(4), 789-791.

Anderson, J. & Olnhausen, K. (1999). Adolescent Self-Esteem: A Foundational Disposition. *Nursing Science Quarterly, 12*(1), 62-67.

Aviles, A. & Helfrich, C.H. (2004). Life Skill Service Needs: Perspectives of Homeless Youth. *Journal of Youth and Adolescence,* 33: 331-338.

Baron, K., Kielhofner, G., Goldhammer, V., & Wolenski, J. (1999). *A User's Manual for the Occupational Self-Assessment (OSA) (Version 1.0).* The Model of Human Occupation Clearinghouse, Department of Occupational Therapy, University of Illinois at Chicago.

Chicago Coalition for the Homeless. *History of Accomplishments.* www.chicagohomeless.org/accomplishments.htm, Accessed March 1, 2005.

Chicago Coalition for the Homeless (2001). Youth on the Streets and on Their Own: Youth Homelessness in Illinois. *A Report by the Chicago Coalition for the Homeless.*

Ensign, J. (2004). Quality of Health Care: The Views of Homeless Youth. *Health Services Research, 39*(4): 695-707.

Ensign, J. & Gittelson, J. (1998). Health and Access to Care: Perspectives of Homeless Youth in Baltimore City, U.S.A. *Social Science Medicine, 47*: 2087-2099.

Gourley, M. (2000). High-Risk Youths Receive OT Intervention. *OT Practice,* May, 9-10.

Greenblatt, M. & Robertson, M. (1993). Life-styles, Adaptive Strategies and Sexual Behavior of Homeless Adolescents. *Hospital, Community Psychiatry, 44*: 1177-1180.

Hammer, H., Finkelhor, D. & Sedlak, A. (2002). Runaway/Throwaway Children: National Estimates and Characteristics. *National Incidence Studies of Missing, Abducted, Runaway, and Throwaway Children.* US Department of Justice. Office of Justice Programs. Office of Juvenile Justice and Delinquency Prevention.

Illinois Poverty Summit. (2004). 2004 Report on Illinois Poverty: Breaking the Cycle of Poverty for Illinois Teens.

Kidd, S. & Scrimenti, K. (2004). Evaluating Child and Youth Homelessness: The Example of New Haven, Connecticut. *Evaluation Review, 28*(4): 325-341.

Klein, J., Woods, A., Wilson, K., Prospero, M., Green, J. & Ringwalt, C. (2000). Homeless and Runaway Youth's Access to Health Care. *Journal of Adolescent Health, 27*(5): 331-339.

Kurtz, P., Lindsey, E., Jarvis, S. & Nackerud, L. (2000). How Runaway and Homeless Youth Navigate Troubled Waters: The Role of Formal and Informal Helpers. *Child and Adolescent Social Work Journal, 17*(5): 381-402.

Levy, J.S. (1998). Homeless Outreach: A Developmental Model. *Psychiatric Rehabilitation Journal, 22*(2):123-131.

Lindsey, E., Kurtz, P., Jarvis, S., Williams, N. & Nackerud, L. (2000). How Runaway and Homeless Youth Navigate Troubled Waters: Personal Strengths and Resources. *Child and Adolescent Social Work Journal, 17*(2): 115-140.

MacLean, M., Embry, L. & Cauce, A. (1999). Homeless Adolescents' Paths to Separation from Family: Comparison of Family Characteristics, Psychological Adjustment and Victimization. *Journal of Community Psychology* (1999) *27*: 179-187.

National Alliance to End Homelessness, Ending Homeless Youth, www.endhomelessness.org/youth/, accessed 08/05/05.

National Alliance to End Homelessness, Youth Homelessness, www.endhomelessness.org/back/YouthFacts.pdf, accessed 1/25/06.

National Coalition for the Homeless, www.nationalhomeless.org, accessed 08/12/05.

Nollan, K.A., Horn, M., Downs, C.A. & Pecora, P.J. (2002). *Ansell-Casey Life Skills Assessment (ACLSA) and Life Skills Guidebook Manual.* Casey Family Programs. Seattle, WA.

Okkema, K. (1993). *Cognition and Perception in the Stroke Patient.* Gaithersburg, MD: Aspen Publication Inc.

Paradise, M. & Cauce, A.M. (2002). Home Street Home: The Interpersonal Dimensions of Adolescent Homelessness. *Analysis of Social Issues and Public Policy, 2*(1): 223-238.

Reeg, B. (2003). The Runaway and Homeless Youth Act and Disconnected Youth, Leave No Youth Behind: Opportunities for Congress to Reach Disconnected

Youth. In Levin-Epstein, J. & Greenburg, M. (Eds.). *Center for Law and Social Policy.*

Reid, P. (1999). Young Homeless People and Service Provision. *Health & Social Care in the Community, 7*(1): 17-24.

Resnick, M.D., Bearman, P.S., Blum, R.W., Bauman, K.E., Harris, K.M., Jones, J., Tabor, J., Beuhring, T., Seiving, R.E., Shew, M., Ireland, M., Bearinger, L.H. & Udry, J.R. (1997). Protecting Adolescents from Harm: Findings from the National Longitudinal Study on Adolescent Health. *Journal of the American Medical Association, 278*(10): 823-832.

Roth, J. & Brooks-Gunn, J. (2000). What Do Adolescents Need for Healthy Development? Implications for Youth Policy. *Social Policy Report, Giving Child and Youth Development Knowledge Away, 14*(1), 3-19.

Schaffner, L. (1998). Searching for Connection: A New Look at Teenaged Runaways. *Adolescence,* 33: 619-628.

Stewart, A., Steinman, M., Cauce, A., Cochran, B., Whitbeck, L. & Hoyt, D. (2004). Victimization and Posttraumatic Stress Disorder Among Homeless Adolescents. *Journal of the American Academy of Child and Adolescent Psychiatry, 43*(3): 325-331.

Vostanis, P. (1999). Child Mental Health Problems. In *Homeless Children: Problems and Needs.* Vostanis, P. & Cumella, S. (Eds.). London: Kingley Publishers.

Vostanis, P., Grattan, E. & Cumella, S. (1998). Mental Health Problems of Homeless Children and Families: Longitudinal Study. *British Medical Journal, 316*: 899-902.

Vostanis, P., Grattan, E., Cumella, S., & Winchester, C. (1997). Psychosocial Functioning of Homeless Children. *Journal of the American Academy of Child & Adolescent Psychiatry, 36*(7): 881-889.

Wrate, R. & Blair, C. (1999). Homeless Adolescents. In *Homeless Children: Problems and Needs.* Vostanis, P. & Cumella, S. (Eds.). London: Kingley Publishers.

doi:10.1300/J003v20n03_07

The After-School Occupations of Homeless Youth: Three Narrative Accounts

Ann E. McDonald, PhD, OTR/L

SUMMARY. This study describes the after-school and weekend time use of young adolescents residing in a temporary shelter for homeless families in Los Angeles County. Data were collected from three individual interviews, focus groups with 24 young adolescents and one-week time use journals. Data were analyzed qualitatively using the constant comparative method. Three narrative profiles were constructed from these data. Emergent themes and concepts describing the occupational

---

Address correspondence to: Ann E. McDonald, 54 N. Lima Street, Sierra Madre, CA 91024 (E-mail: annandlily@msn.com).

This paper addresses the diverse ways in which homeless youth perceive their occupational engagement and its relationship to personal health in the after-school hours. It was condensed from research conducted in partial fulfillment of the requirement for the degree of Doctor of Philosophy in Occupational Science from the University of Southern California, Los Angeles.

This study was partially funded by a Leadership Training Grant from the Bureau of Maternal and Child Health and a Wilma West Scholarship from the American Occupational Therapy Foundation (AOTF).

The author wishes to acknowledge the invaluable guidance from her chairperson, Dr. Ruth Zemke, and members of her dissertation committee: Dr. Diane Parham and Dr. Jacquelyn McCroskey.

[Haworth co-indexing entry note]: "The After-School Occupations of Homeless Youth: Three Narrative Accounts." McDonald, Ann E. Co-published simultaneously in *Occupational Therapy in Health Care* (The Haworth Press, Inc.) Vol. 20, No. 3/4, 2006, pp. 115-133; and: *Homelessness in America: Perspectives, Characterizations, and Considerations for Occupational Therapy* (ed: Kathleen Swenson Miller, Georgiana L. Herzberg, and Sharon A. Ray) The Haworth Press, Inc., 2006, pp. 115-133. Single or multiple copies of this article are available for a fee from The Haworth Document Delivery Service [1-800-HAWORTH, 9:00 a.m. - 5:00 p.m. (EST). E-mail address: docdelivery@haworthpress.com].

Available online at http://othc.haworthpress.com
© 2006 by The Haworth Press, Inc. All rights reserved.
doi:10.1300/J003v20n03_08

participation of young adolescents during the non-school hours were summarized into three major concepts. These were the following: (a) Occupational Necessity: Social Intensity; (b) Boredom and Shelter Living: Occupational Advantages and Disadvantages; and, (c) Designing a Life: Taking Control. Implications for occupational science, occupational therapy, and public policy were identified with relevant recommendations. doi:10.1300/J003v20n03_08 *[Article copies available for a fee from The Haworth Document Delivery Service: 1-800-HAWORTH. E-mail address: <docdelivery@haworthpress.com> Website: <http://www.HaworthPress.com>* *© 2006 by The Haworth Press, Inc. All rights reserved.]*

KEYWORDS. Homeless youth, health, occupation building

BACKGROUND OF THE PROBLEM

Most Americans most likely never experience homelessness, but in the recent aftermath of Hurricane Katrina we are witnessing first-hand accounts of what it means to lose the stability of shelter, food, community life, and even predictable daily routines. Individuals who were thrust into homelessness now must deal with the multiple demands of finding housing, employment, and new ways to meet their basic physical and social-emotional needs. Prior to this catastrophic event, many of these families were living at or below the poverty line but did not yet meet the criteria for homelessness.

Families are the fastest growing segment of the homeless population, accounting for 40% of the nation's homeless. Single women with children comprise approximately 85% of homeless families. Studies on homelessness show homeless families often do not experience safety, stability, or good health outcomes. Chronic unemployment, underemployment, poor health and nutrition, drug and alcohol abuse, domestic violence, and incarceration are common in homeless families and are often precursors to homelessness. Homeless youth are at an increased risk for developing physical, learning, and mental health problems (Committee on Community Health Services, 2005).

Frequent school changes, poor attendance, and a two-fold increase in repeating a grade and being suspended are all common characteristics for homeless youth. Learning problems such as speech delays and reading difficulties are twice as common for homeless youth when compared with other non-homeless children (National Center for Homeless Education, 2006; The Better Homes Fund, 1999). Nearly one-third of school age children who are homeless have at least one major mental disorder, such as anxiety, depression, or withdrawal. However, less than one third of these children are reported to receive any treatment. In addition, poor nutritional status, low self-esteem, and a greater risk of contracting AIDS or HIV-related illnesses are some of the major health risks facing homeless youth today (National Coalition for the Homeless, 2005).

RATIONALE FOR STUDY

Less is known in the literature about the self-reported occupational pursuits of homeless youth during non-school hours and the relationship between the youth's perceived personal health and occupational choices. The occupational choices made by the young adolescent, especially during the non-school hours, appear closely related to the negative or positive health outcomes in the youth's present, and possibly, future (National Mental Health Association, 2006; Office of the Surgeon General, 1996; 2002).

Occupational choice refers to the selection of occupations, activities or daily pursuits that are personally and culturally meaningful (Zemke & Clark, 1996). Occupational scientists are interested in how individuals choose to engage or not engage in certain occupations, and the relationship between occupation and health. Occupational scientists are also interested in how individuals ascribe meaning to time use and occupation and, consequently, how occupation promotes health and adaptation (Zemke & Clark).

Identifying and describing the types of after-school occupations, patterns of time use, and the meanings of these choices by young adolescents would assist social scientists and policymakers, including occupational scientists and occupational therapists, with interpreting behaviors as well as with guiding the development of after-school programs in the community (Jackson & Arbesman, 2005). Those behaviors believed to confer positive health benefits are identified in this study as health-enhancing occupations while those believed detrimental are identified as health-compromising occupations (Elliott, 1993).

RESEARCH DESIGN

This study describes the after-school and weekend time use of young adolescents (ages 10 to 14) who reside in a temporary shelter with their families. The data include excerpts from individual interviews, focus groups, and one-week time use journals. Specifically, three narrative profiles were developed from three of the 24 participants in this study. These profiles were the result of synthesis of data obtained from the verbal interviews and written records. The focus group sessions comprised approximately four children, with boys and girls in separate groups. Each group met two to three times, one week apart. Thus, over the course of a year-and-a-half, four focus groups of girls and three focus groups of boys were interviewed in a semi-structured format in order to learn how youths used and perceived their time use during the non-school hours. In addition, one-week time use journals were completed by all of the participants and were utilized to identify self-reported activities and subjective reports of time use. Data compiled from all participants in focus groups and participants' time use journals were used to answer the research questions guiding this study.

Participants were in families of low socioeconomic minority backgrounds who met the definition for being homeless. The 24 participants were comprised of 13 females and 11 males with twice as many Latinos as African-Americans. The study was conducted at a temporary homeless shelter in Southern California, located on the grounds of a maximum security psychiatric hospital. The high security areas of the hospital, surrounded by barbed wire, are visible from the backyard of the shelter. The perceived influence of the surrounding environment is reported in the descriptive narratives.

The research questions chosen to guide this inquiry into the daily lives of homeless youth were the following: (1) What occupations and occupational routines do homeless adolescents report engaging in after school and on the weekends? (2) What meanings do homeless adolescents assign to their after-school occupations and time use during non-school hours? (3) What meanings do homeless adolescents assign to personal health and its relationship to occupational engagement? (4) What are other potential influences on time use during the non-school hours?

DATA ANALYSIS AND INTERPRETATION

Data collected from the one-week journal records, the complete transcripts from the focus groups and individual interviews were used to answer the research questions. Qualitative data analysis and interpretation were used to describe the occupational time use of the participants in this study. Emerging themes and any unexpected themes from the data were identified using the constant comparative method (Strauss & Corbin,

1998). All the data were coded by the researcher into the following emergent themes or initial categories: (1) Obligatory Occupations, (2) Voluntary Occupations, (3) Occupational Routines and Boredom, (4) Personal Health and Occupation, and (5) Variables Influencing Time Use.

For the purposes of this study, data from these emergent themes were used to answer the research questions and, with further analysis, led to the development of the three personal narratives and were summarized into three major concepts. These three concepts were the following: (1) Occupational Necessity: Social Intensity, (2) Boredom and Shelter Living: Occupational Advantages and Disadvantages, and (3) Designing a Life: Taking Control. These major concepts help elucidate the occupational nature of the participants during the non-school hours.

The reliability and validity of these methods were based on three procedures described by Krefting (1990). *First*, the credibility of the research process was based on the investigator's personal reflections on the dynamic relationship with the participants and the process through which meanings were produced and information was framed or interpreted. *Second*, the reoccurrence of general emergent themes in the data was identified that adequately represented the experiences reported by youth as verified by member checking. In addition, a second reviewer of the written transcripts acted as a content expert to provide further identification and interpretation of emerging categories and themes. This level of analysis provided narrative descriptions to explore not only what youths reported doing but also what meanings were attributed to their occupational engagement. *Third*, while the actual use of the participant's time may not always be known, the consistency of the participant's report over time and in different formats (i.e., time use journals, focus groups, individual interviews) was used to serve as a check and add rigor to the study. This multi-method process, also known as triangulation, increased the credibility, dependability, and confirmability of the data in the study.

NARRATIVE PROFILES

The three narrative profiles provide phenomenological or personal meanings youths attributed to their after-school time use and how youths knowingly or unknowingly utilized different resources and modes of adapting to life in the homeless shelter. The first profile summarizes "Mary's" responses. Her narrative theme seemed to be best described by her statement during one group, "I am making the best of it."

Mary's Story: "Making the Best of It"

Mary, a 10-year-old Latina, described some of her favorite after-school play activities as "playing pirates or school" or having a pumpkin carving contest. When asked what activity she did after school that made her physically feel good, she stated, "running and playing basketball because it makes me feel excited inside and like . . . freedom." I also asked her to tell me about a favorite time she had after school. She described how happy she was when her mother picked her up from school and "everyone saw my mom for the first time." She expressed how much she enjoyed "cuddling up" with her mom in the evenings before bedtime. Mary appeared to crave any time she had with her mother due to her mother's seven day work week. Mary's affect often appeared flat or constrained when she was in child care after school, but she reported in her journal that she felt "OK" at the time. She also reported feeling "very happy" when her mother arrived home and they ate dinner together.

Despite having the desire to play games typical of 10-year-old girls, Mary also showed a maturity beyond her years. One example of this maturity was observed in response to my question to the group, "Did anyone want to write in their journal that they were having fun even if they weren't?" Mary replied, "No, well, I TRY to make it fun everyday." She also described how much her mother helped her cope with boredom at the shelter. She stated, "When it was a boring time, my mom tried to make the best of it. She tried to give us games or tell us how to play a dice game. She always tried to make the best out of it." She also described her struggles in dealing with the many restrictions on her time: "Like on the weekend I'm more free to do things and during the week it's like I'm trapped. You know, I have to stay in my room. We can't go out. Then my weekends I have all free and I feel more emotionally happy and I could do more things."

The majority of Mary's responses appeared closely related to her emotional or subjective experience of boredom, frustration, and sadness while living at the shelter. For example, her interpretation of the words "personal health" was both insightful for her age and revealed some of the inner resources she appeared to be utilizing in constructing a lifestyle that met her emotional needs and consequent occupational behavior. Mary stated, "To me [personal health] means to keep yourself strong. You need to have like time for yourself . . . and someone to talk to because if you just keep your things inside they'll just stay there . . . like it affects your health and you're really sad and angry. It makes you feel . . . like you're not breathing. That you're so mad 'cause you're not telling anybody about it."

Mary also vividly described the change in her emotion from feeling "trapped" during the week at the shelter to the weekends when "they finally open up the gates and we're free."

However, when asked how she would feel when she left the shelter, Mary expressed some ambivalence and said, "I think I would feel more alone . . . 'cause here I'm used to the noise and [there] it'll be so quiet . . . I would be totally different, 'cause here it's like I go to child care. I have to walk straight home but [in the future] I would go to my friend's house, do my homework, then I'll play baseball. Then I'll do a lot of things and get my mind off my homework."

Mary did not mention participating in any high-risk activities (e.g., fighting or drug use) but instead focused on the importance of being with friends and family. Her story emphasized her perseverance in finding ways to adapt to her present living situation. She appeared to use her inner resources of being optimistic and focusing on the positive aspects of her present life situation, over which she appeared to have little control. She also reported seeking out extra-personal resources such as engagement in social occupations to help her deal with boredom and frustration. Talking with friends, her mother, as well as the counselor were all adaptive strategies she used to help her deal with stressful situations at the shelter.

Mimi's Story: "If I Get Bored My Mom Knows I'll Do Something!"

While Mary's story is one of perseverance and adaptation, other girls were much less able to problem-solve on how to deal with their stress and seek out resources to help their situation. Mimi was a Latina, 12 years old going on 20, figuratively speaking. Her interviews were frequently accounts of how mad and bored she was at the shelter. She emphatically described how angry she would become by saying, "If I get mad, I like throw a tornado! I remember one time I tried to hit my grandma 'cause I was so mad . . . but I don't get mad fast." During the discussion on weekend time use, she matter-of-factly described how she almost burned down her grandmother's house because she was so bored. She stated how upset she was because she had to spend "a whole weekend with my grandma . . . who I think is really, really boring."

Mimi had much difficulty identifying any activities she could do while staying with her grandmother for the weekend, even though in the group she reported to like listening to music, writing, and watching TV. Instead, she stated, "My grandma don't have no activities there. She lives in East L.A. and like she always has a bunch of Cholos over there and there's nothing to do there. All I could do is like make trouble . . . there's nothing but trouble over there." Mimi stated she would never cause trouble at her grandmother's house again because "my mom whipped my butt." Shortly later she replied, "If I get really bored my mom knows I will do something."

When asked to describe a typical day after school, she named each activity as if reading a monotonous list. She said, "I do my homework, watch TV, then play the game, go and eat, and then come back in here [inside the shelter]." She also remarked that she frequently talked to another girl in the group with whom she often stayed up late at night playing games in each other's rooms. I asked her if that was alright with her mother. She explained that, as long as her mother got her sleep, her mother didn't care if she wanted to stay up late.

Even time spent alone after school was described with apathy. "It's boring 'cause you're all by yourself and you don't know what to do. For me, sometimes it's not boring. It's like I can yell my head off and nobody will care." This latter statement appeared to reflect her inner turmoil of not feeling heard or cared about. She said her mother let her do some of the activities she wanted to do (e.g., staying up late), but it was interesting to note that she also said her mother "didn't care" about what she did. She also remarked that her mother was always nagging at her and she couldn't do her homework over her mother's voice. In contrast to Mary, Mimi reported a high degree of tension in her daily interactions with her mother.

Mimi did report feeling close to her father who did not live near the shelter. She stated, "I like going to my dad's 'cause he's like the 'out' kind of person, unless there's football on TV–then we won't go nowhere. But he takes us fishing, and he'll drop us off somewhere, wherever. He took us to the Santa Monica Pier, swimming, mountain climbing . . . he took us a lot of places." She stated she could no longer do any of those activities with her dad since she came to the shelter because he now lived further away. Losing valued time with her father was also another apparent loss or stressor for Mimi since coming to the shelter.

John's Story: "I Run, Eat, and Play: I'm My Own Boy."

John is a 13-year-old African-American male whose story is not necessarily typical of all boys in this study, but it does describe the commonly found reports of feeling trapped and wanting freedom away from the shelter. At the time of the interview, he reported he had been with his family at the shelter for six months. He explained how he dealt with life at the shelter and on the weekends, as well as how he used to spend his after-school time and what he hoped for the future.

During the interview, John matter-of-factly explained his typical after-school routine. This included catching the bus home, doing five minutes of homework, eating dinner, taking a shower, ironing his clothes, and getting ready for school the next day. When asked what he liked to do for fun after school at the shelter, he said, "I'm playing with my sisters . . . we play outside . . . tag, swinging contest [on swings], everything." He stated he used to play football after school and he wished he could do that now, but he couldn't because he had to catch the bus home. He also said his typical routine used to involve staying longer at school or going home and then coming right back to school. After- school activities used to include running track, playing basketball, going to dances, having water balloon fights, and "a whole lot of stuff."

John also talked about having a lot of friends at school. When asked if he could bring any of his friends to the shelter, he said, "No, 'cause you can't have company in here." His mother would sometimes take him to the store or to see his uncle. I asked him if he had people to talk to when he needed to and he replied, "Yeah, all the time. We talk about important stuff and we just be talking and talking." Talking, he reported, was important for having good health because, "like you just talk, you let the air out." His response was similar to Mary's comment on ". . . not keeping your bad feelings inside." Like Mary, he also mentioned the importance of exercise to "stay strong" and "don't do smoking or nothing like that."

When asked if he had time for himself at the shelter, he stated, "I'm by myself with all my sisters. Like we be here sometimes, my sisters be like in over there watching a movie; my mom be talking on the phone. So I be in there [the bedroom] by myself laying down watching TV." I asked if being alone also meant getting to do what he wanted to do and he said, "Right, because I'm my own boy." This latter comment also reflected John's separateness from his family, although he appeared emotionally very close to them. More important, was his self-described sense of becoming in charge of his world.

Compared to other participants, John was given more freedom on the weekends. For example, his mother gave him permission to visit a friend from his old neighborhood. He was allowed to take a bus over to his friend's house about 30 minutes away and would call his mother after he arrived. Taking the bus alone (although not approved by the shelter staff) was one way John was able to develop his sense of responsibility and earn a privilege based on his behavior following the rules set by his mother. John appeared to be using a variety of resources to help him cope with living in the shelter. This included his experience with past occupations to construct present occupations or activities that were adaptive in helping him adjust to all the restrictions imposed by the shelter.

The most important players in his story were, first and foremost, his family, especially his mother and sisters. Friendships from the past and present were also an important resource to him. He was able to develop friendships at his new school within the six months he lived at the shelter. He also described being well-liked by others at school, even though he exaggerated a little by calling the whole school his "friend."

SUMMARY OF NARRATIVE PROFILES

Although their subjective experience of occupational performance was not always known to the investigator, youths in this study provided many examples of their past and present occupational behavior, including the importance of these experiences in their lives. The lived experiences shared by these youths were interpreted by the investigator using the following three concepts to summarize their occupational nature.

Occupational Necessity: Social Intensity

Spending time with family or friends was, in almost all reports from the participants in this study, a primary occupation during non-school hours. The close relationship youths reported between their perceptions of positive emotional health and participation in social occupations was found in the majority of their interviews and journal reports. The importance of having a friend focused on the need for companionship and understanding. Friends were primarily described by girls as important for "having someone to talk to" about one's problems and concerns, while boys talked more about having friends "to hang out with."

Girls focused much of their discussion of discretionary time use on the importance of being with their friends. Boys more often described friends by their utilitarian value: that is, a necessary part of an activity they wanted to perform after school. For example, instead of talking to friends about their "problems or concerns" as reported by the girls, boys described wanting to participate in informal sports or other activities such as "playing basketball" and "going to the beach and park with friends."

Friends from previous neighborhoods and schools were also frequently mentioned as being missed. Like John, a few children reported being able to see friends on the weekend, but this was not possible for many due to the extended distance from their previous community and transportation problems. In addition, some youths were too embarrassed to tell their friends that they now lived in a shelter. The loss of past friendships and break-up of families so often experienced by these youths seemed to give them an impetus to form new relationships with other children at the shelter in the same situation.

In this study, feelings of happiness and contentment were more closely associated with social occupations with friends and family than when activities were performed alone. Although most youths in this study did not verbalize their reasons for wanting to spend time with their parent(s), they often wrote in their journals how "happy" they were spending time with them. This finding was also supported by Rutter's (1985, 1993) research that identified resiliency or protective factors associated with positive health outcomes for children. Specifically, positive experiences of secure relationships were strongly associated with positive physical and mental health. However, Rutter did not specifically identify engagement in personally meaningful occupations as contributing to resiliency. This finding of the importance of engagement in meaningful occupation during the non-school hours and perceived positive health by homeless youth is addressed in the next sections.

Boredom and Shelter Living: Occupational Advantages and Disadvantages

The experience of living at the shelter was described by the majority of the participants as "boring," as if they were "trapped" or "locked up" in a prison under constant surveillance by adults. The meanings young adolescents attributed to this spatial constraint on their daily occupational pursuits are summed up with this prison metaphor. The restriction of their physical movement since arriving at the shelter seemed to be very upsetting since they reported having more freedom in the past in deciding how they would spend their after-school time. One child summed up the feelings of most youths by saying, "We need our space too!"

It was not surprising to this investigator that participants reported feeling bored with their after-school routines. Over a two-and-a-half year period I observed the types of activities offered by the shelter. The weekly routine was invariably the same unless a parent had given approval to his or her child to attend certain after-school activities (e.g., drill team, YMCA). The majority of the children returned home to the shelter and reported having no freedom to go anywhere, except to child care or with their parents. Thus, the routine was fairly predictable and typically involved the following sequence: doing some errands with their parents or staying at the shelter with other children playing games in child care, doing homework, doing simple chores, eating dinner, watching television, and then going to bed. Occasionally, individual counseling, art therapy, and tutoring were available to the children.

Occupational Advantages of Boredom

An occupational advantage for living at the shelter was the predictability in routine that offered a safe, although "boring," haven away from their previous home environment that often included a chaotic living situation with domestic violence, drug abuse, loss of employment, disability, or other precursors to homelessness. Many participants attributed their feelings of boredom, sadness, and frustration as due to the many restrictions placed on their behavior at the shelter instead of to other plausible reasons related to their homelessness. While it was apparent that there were many restrictions on families, there was a sense of safety and predictability many families had not experienced consistently in their lives.

Youths in this study also described how they developed friendships quickly in order to "do something" and seemed for a moment to forget their pervasive sense of boredom. Occupational routines that included the development of a peer network to help cope with the loss of previous friendships appeared necessary for these youths to cope with their present situation. Thus, boredom was the impetus to develop and engage in social occupations that were incorporated into everyday routines familiar to them from their past living situation. These social routines appeared to provide the continuity youths needed in their daily life path and helped them to create, or recreate, themselves as young adolescents seeking some degree of autonomy in the daily occupations they chose to engage, or not engage in, during the non-school hours.

Occupational Disadvantages of Boredom

Occupational disadvantages of boredom for some youths included a perceived loss of control resulting in a need to express one's frustration by acting out or possibly participating in health-compromising occupations. For example, Mimi proclaimed to the group she would "do something" (referring to her past episode of getting into trouble) if she became very bored. Other youths did not express this extreme response to feeling bored, but did talk about the frustration they felt being under constant adult supervision.

One girl described how difficult it was to wake up her mother because she was not allowed to walk down the hall by herself to go to the bathroom. She stated, "You feel like you're her dog or something!" (Others in the group nodded in agreement.) This analogy depicted the low self-esteem that appeared to be the result of the message youths felt was conveyed to them by the rules of the shelter environment; You are not trustworthy to be on your own and, sadly, not even human! These examples portray how the personal identity and life path were being constructed for some of these youths.

The majority of children in this study appeared to have found different ways of creatively coping with their boredom in the present, as well as simultaneously planning their future occupational lives outside the shelter. Boredom related to a highly supervised setting with few desirable occupational choices may increase the risk of health-compromising behaviors for some youths but also may confer health benefits for others and provide the impetus for youths to engage in adaptive behaviors such as creative occupation-making.

Designing a Life: Taking Control

The three personal narratives reported above demonstrated how teens in different circumstances developed different strategies to deal with their present situation and plan for future occupations. These narrative profiles lend support for the basic assumptions of occupational science. These include the following: (1) engagement in meaningful occupation is essential to health; (2) the recursive relationship between occupation and narrative shapes personal identity, and (3) humans are most true to themselves when they are engaged in meaningful and satisfying occupation (Clark, 1997). Occupations are also described by occupational scientists as having an unfolding nature influenced by the individual and the setting. Thus, occupations are not considered equally meaningful and can vary depending on one's values, hopes, experiences, objectives, and life narratives (Mandel, Jackson, Zemke, Nelson, & Clark, 1999).

Mary's optimistic attitude to "make the best of it" in the present moment appeared to be an adaptive strategy she used to deal with the present, as well as to plan for her future occupational time use. She described how she felt emotionally close to her mother who helped her deal with boredom at the shelter. Her desires for close emotional and physical contact with her mother, close friendships to discuss her feelings, and a variety of after-school activities with friends indicate her future construction of personally meaningful occupations based on a strong value of being emotionally connected to others. Her occupational choices were shaped by these desires in her present situation at the shelter as she often talked about enjoying structured activities that were "interesting" in child care (e.g., going to the movies, being in a club).

However, Mary also had somatic complaints (i.e., headaches) when doing homework and felt bored when her mother was not present. She was observed, at times, during child-care activities to be withdrawn and having a flat affect. Her comments that there were not enough interesting activities in child care could be, in part, interpreted to mean she had little control over her occupational choices. She was not known to participate in any observable health-compromising behaviors, but she appeared to be experiencing depression over her present situation.

Mary demonstrated several resiliency factors. Specifically, I observed her to have a style of acting rather than reacting, self-efficacy and problem solving, positive experiences of successful relationships, and qualities engendering a positive response from others. Engagement in personally meaningful occupations also appears to be a resiliency factor for Mary. The complexity of the relationships between protective mechanisms and the multiple contexts and domains within which these occur need to be better understood for at-risk youth (Blum, McNeely, & Nonnemaker, 2002). However, it appears evident that Mary's ability to access extra and intra-personal resources to find ways to engage in occupations with some degree of choice and social engagement were protective mechanisms within the shelter environment. Thus, Mary's resiliency in the face of adverse circumstances included occupational choices that seemed to be leaning towards positive health outcomes and meeting her occupational needs for the future.

Likewise, John described several strategies that were successful for him in meeting his occupational needs. He described how he had befriended peers at his new school. He also emphasized the enjoyment he felt traveling by himself to visit a friend from his old neighborhood. He sought assistance doing homework from his family and enjoyed a variety of leisure activities.

In addition, John talked about having time on his own after dinner even with his family present. His statement, "I'm my own boy," was a proud response to how he felt about his experiences living at the shelter with his family. John's engagement in meaningful occupations seemed to be shaped by his past experiences in a similar after- school routine, which included spending time with his family and friends, doing his chores and homework, and being on his own. His present occupational pursuits appeared not only adaptive in a new setting but also continued to reinforce his self-identity; that is, being a young male teen with increasing responsibility and a sense of competency in social relationships. This increased efficacy appeared to lead to his continued success in making new friends and in taking on greater responsibilities to obtain some of his desired occupations (i.e., seeing friends from his past neighborhood).

In terms of the relationship between John's occupational engagement and his health, his self-perceptions were that he had good health because he exercised to "stay strong," "didn't do smoking or nothing like that," and talked to his friends to "just let the air out." His self-report was validated only to the extent that he was not known to have any reported difficulties in getting along with others in the shelter or at school. Although he had many learning difficulties, he did not seem to be focused on these deficits but, instead, described his present situation as "alright" and expressed hope for his future. John's reported participation in a variety of personally meaningful after- school and weekend occupations seemed to be a major resiliency factor that helped him to adapt to his present situation and prepare him for a future of more health-enhancing occupations.

Finally, Mimi's reports of feeling so bored that she knew she would get into trouble suggested she had few desirable occupations to participate in after school or on the weekends. She described social activities away from the shelter as the most enjoyable but she could not think of anything enjoyable to do at the shelter except talking to one of her friends. Mimi also expressed far fewer positive remarks and more negative comments than John and Mary when discussing how she felt about living at the shelter. In addition, she reported frequent participation in fights at school and feeling ambivalent about her relationship with her mother.

Mimi's self-reported frequency of participation in health-compromising occupations was, not surprisingly, much higher than any other participant, except perhaps her brother. Her approach in dealing with her present situation was to demonstrate a tough, bravado image, one she likely relied upon in the past when dealing with difficult aspects in her life. Mimi's desire for future occupations included activities that other girls in the group also reported wanting to do more (i.e., being in a club, meeting at the mall, going to the movies or shopping–ultimately, being away from the shelter with friends). Like Mary, she also desired to have more time with one of her parents (i.e., her father). Mimi did not seem to have a close relationship with her mother nor with many other children at the shelter. She talked about being thought of as a "weirdo" by other children at school and that nobody really listened to her. Her self-report of feeling rejected, isolated, bored, and angry is cause for concern not only for her poor self-esteem and future personal identity, but also for her high risk of future involvement in health-compromising occupations (given her past history and her immediate stressors from being homeless).

Mimi did not appear to obtain much satisfaction from her occupational routines at the shelter but she did attempt to find some activities that were positive in helping her participate in health-enhancing occupations (e.g., joining a club, finding supportive friendships). Her personal identity was being shaped by a strong need for control in her perceived out-of-control lifestyle. The question for all children like Mimi who are facing a similar situation is this: What will determine their ability to choose health-enhancing versus health-compromising occupations? The answer to this question, I believe, depends on the presence of a significant caring adult who will be available to help at-risk youth find satisfying and meaningful occupations.

Thus, the above three narrative profiles were presented with additional data sources from the findings in an unpublished dissertation (McDonald, 2001) to support the basic assumptions of occupational science and provide information about some of the issues facing the everyday lives of children residing in a homeless shelter during the non-school hours. The pragmatic value for this research is to chart the way in which public policy and social service providers, including occupational therapy, can address some of the concerns expressed by these young adolescents by guiding them in their present and future occupational pursuits.

Policy and Program Recommendations

Below are recommendations by which community or shelter after-school programs could meet the occupational needs of youth from vulnerable backgrounds:

1. On a local level, policymakers should consider ways to ease access and availability of publicly-funded after-school programs for homeless and other low-income youths residing in their communities, including transportation to programs if needed.
2. After-school programs should provide youths a wide array of activities, including significant input and buy-in from the youths themselves. Allowing youths to be more autonomous from adults in their occupational choices and to problem-solve with consultation by an adult mentor may help them own the process of their occupational engagement and express their emerging sense of self.
3. After-school programs need to include physical activities involving structured and unstructured sports and leisure activities. To

their credit, many after-school programs do attempt to provide such activities. However, the importance of these activities to the youth's emotional well-being needs to be taken into greater consideration. As youths in this study so clearly described, after-school occupations that include vigorous activity provide them with a sense of well-being and a socially acceptable means to help them alleviate some of the stress in their daily lives.

Participation in various types of sports activities, especially team sports, and active unstructured leisure activities (e.g., bike riding) were mentioned by both girls and boys as very desirable after-school activities. However, there was often not enough space to participate in these activities at the shelter or at safe places with adequate equipment within the community. Participation in structured and unstructured sports activities was explicitly reported by all youth as helping them deal with their frustrations in their daily lives and, in turn, providing them with physical and mental health benefits.

4. Occupational therapists can play a vital role as service providers within homeless shelters for families with children. An untapped arena for occupational therapy intervention was discovered with the findings from this research; that is, homeless adolescents were adamant about having their individual needs met for more choices of interesting after-school activities, more autonomy in their use of time after school, and more time to spend with friends and a significant adult. Occupational therapists can play a vital role in assisting homeless and at-risk youths by problem-solving how to redesign their after-school time use and finding creative solutions to deal with boredom and violence within their community. Participation in special interests as well as exposure to new and different occupational choices would provide youths with a stronger sense of personal identity as "doers"; that is, seeking new ways to learn about their potential and be true to their emerging self.

In summary, this study highlights how homeless youths engage in occupation building when faced with the loss of familiar routines and valued occupations. Youths in this study constructed new and familiar routines based on a complex relationship between extra-personal and intra-personal influences and resources. Although it was beyond the present scope to provide an in-depth analysis of these relationships, these data provide the impetus for further research and program recommendations.

Specifically, research on a larger scale is needed to determine if similar findings emerge in other groups of at-risk youth as well as to identify longitudinal trends in time use and how occupational routines are related to future health-compromising and health-enhancing lifestyles. These findings would also provide clarity for specific recommendations for policymakers and implementation of outcomes-based after-school programs. Despite known limitations, the present study sets the stage for the creative implementation of occupational therapy programs in a novel practice arena.

REFERENCES

Blum, R. W., McNeely, C., & Nonnemaker, J. (2002). Vulnerability, risk, and protection. *Journal of Adolescent Health 31,* Suppl. 1, pp. 28-39.

Clark, F. (1997). Appendix III: Occupational science. In P. Crist & C. B. Royeen, *Infusing occupation into practice: Comparison of three clinical approaches in occupational therapy* (pp. 101-111). Bethesda, MD: The American Occupational Therapy Association, Inc.

Committee on Community Health Services (2005). Providing care for immigrant, homeless, and migrant children. *Pediatrics 115*, 1095-1100.

Elliott, D. S. (1993). Health enhancing and health compromising lifestyles. In S. G. Millstein, A. C. Petersen, & E. O. Nightingale (Eds.), *Promoting the health of adolescents* (pp. 119-145). New York: Oxford University Press.

Jackson, L., & Arbesman, M. (Eds.) (2005). *Occupational therapy practice guidelines for children with behavioral and psychosocial needs.* Bethesda, MD: The AOTA Press.

Krefting, L. (1990). Rigor in qualitative research. *American Journal of Occupational Therapy 45*, 214-222.

Mandel, D. R., Jackson, J. M., Zemke, R., Nelson, L., & Clark, F. (1999). *Lifestyle redesign: Implementing the well elderly program.* Bethesda, MD: The American Occupational Therapy Association (AOTA), Bethesda, MD: The AOTA Press.

McDonald, A. (2001). *The after school occupations of homeless youth: Implications for occupational science, occupational therapy & public policy.* Unpublished doctoral dissertation, University of Southern California, Los Angeles.

National Center for Homeless Education (2006). *Homeless in America: A children's story.* [On line]. Available: http://serve.org/nche.

National Mental Health Association (2006). *Fact sheet on children and homelessness* [On line]. Available: http://www.nmha.org/homeless.html.

Office of the Surgeon General (1996). *Physical activity and health: A report of the surgeon general.* Available: http://www.cdc.gov/nccdphp/sgr/content.html.

Office of the Surgeon General (2002). *Youth violence: A report of the surgeon general* [On line]. Available: http://www.cdc.gov/nccdphp/sgr/content/html.

Rutter, M. (1985). Resilience in the face of adversity: Protective factors and resistance to psychiatric disorder. *British Journal of Psychiatry 147*, 598-611.

Rutter, M. (1993). Resilience: Some conceptual considerations. *Journal of Adolescent Health 14*, 626-631.

Strauss, A., & Corbin, J. (1998). *Basis of qualitative research techniques and procedures for developing grounded theory* (2nd Ed.). Thousand Oaks, CA: Sage Publications.

The Better Homes Fund (1999). *America's homeless children: New outcasts.* Public policy report (number 99-63630). Available from The Better Homes Fund, 181 Wells Avenue, Newton, MA. 02549-3344.

Zemke, R., & Clark, F. A. (Eds.) (1996). *Occupational science: The evolving discipline.* Philadelphia: F. A. Davis Co.

doi:10.1300/J003v20n03_08

APPLICATION

Assessing the Occupational Performance Priorities of People Who Are Homeless

Jaime Phillip Muñoz, PhD, OTR, FAOTA
Teressa Garcia, BS
Joy Lisak, BA
Diana Reichenbach, MOT, OTR/L

Jaime Phillip Muñoz, Assistant Professor, Teressa Garcia, Graduate Student, and Joy Lisak, Graduate Student, are affiliated with Duquesne University, Department of Occupational Therapy. Diana Reichenbach is Program Director, Project Employ, Bethlehem Haven, Pittsburgh, PA.

Address correspondence to: Jaime Phillip Muñoz, Assistant Professor, Duquesne University, Department of Occupational Therapy, 219 Health Science Building, Pittsburgh, PA 15282 (E-mail: munoz@duq.edu).

The authors are indebted to the following individuals who are just a few of the many collaborators whose support has ensured the success of Project Employ: Marilyn Sullivan, Bethlehem Haven Executive Director, Sara Dix, Occupational Therapist, Project Employ, Connie Lewski, Employment Specialist, Project Employ, Nicole Ford, Bethlehem Haven Data Base Manager, Anne Marie Witchger Hansen, Instructor, Duquesne University, and Dr. Patricia Crist, Professor and Chair of the Department of Occupational Therapy at Duquesne University.

[Haworth co-indexing entry note]: "Assessing the Occupational Performance Priorities of People Who Are Homeless." Muñoz, Jaime Phillip et al. Co-published simultaneously in *Occupational Therapy in Health Care* (The Haworth Press, Inc.) Vol. 20, No. 3/4, 2006, pp. 135-148; and: *Homelessness in America: Perspectives, Characterizations, and Considerations for Occupational Therapy* (ed: Kathleen Swenson Miller, Georgiana L. Herzberg, and Sharon A. Ray) The Haworth Press, Inc., 2006, pp. 135-148. Single or multiple copies of this article are available for a fee from The Haworth Document Delivery Service [1-800-HAWORTH, 9:00 a.m. - 5:00 p.m. (EST). E-mail address: docdelivery@haworthpress.com].

Available online at http://othc.haworthpress.com
© 2006 by The Haworth Press, Inc. All rights reserved.
doi:10.1300/J003v20n03_09

SUMMARY. This study examined retrospective data for 65 participants enrolled in an occupational therapy supportive employment program. The Canadian Occupational Performance Measure (COPM) was used to identify self-perceived occupational performance problems specific to this population. Over half of the identified problems fell in the self-care domain (59%), about one-third (31%) were in the productivity domain and the final 10% were in the leisure domain. Narrative analysis of verbatim goals suggests that these individuals identified different types of self-care and productivity problems than samples in previous studies. The results of this study indicate that the COPM can facilitate person-centered, culturally responsive assessment with individuals who are homeless. doi:10.1300/J003v20n03_09 *[Article copies available for a fee from The Haworth Document Delivery Service: 1-800-HAWORTH. E-mail address: <docdelivery@haworthpress.com> Website: <http://www.HaworthPress.com>* *© 2006 by The Haworth Press, Inc. All rights reserved.]*

KEYWORDS. COPM, homelessness, culturally responsive assessment

A lack of housing is only one dimension of the homeless experience. There are a number of complex, interrelated factors that contribute to homelessness including a lack of education, inadequate and inconsistent access to health care (O'Toole & Withers, 1998), domestic violence (National Coalition for the Homeless, 2002), unemployment, mental illness (Gonzalez & Rosenheck, 2002; Toro & Warren, 1999) and addiction (Steinhaus, Harley, & Rogers, 2004). Unemployment, poverty, and social stigma are also common experiences of those without a home (Hwang, 2001).

Occupational therapists are increasingly demonstrating how societal problems such as poverty, addiction, violence or chronic homelessness can be addressed from an occupational perspective (Kronenberg, Algado, & Pollard, 2005). Over the past several years, descriptions of community-university partnerships that demonstrate how occupational therapists are well-suited to provide core services at homeless shelters have appeared in the professional literature (Finlayson, Baker, Rodman, & Herzberg, 2002; Muñoz, Reichenbach, & Hansen, 2005; Tryssenaar, Jones, & Lee, 1999). Collectively, these authors give voice to the complex set of intervention challenges presented by persons who are homeless. Addressing these challenges requires that practitioners employ person-centered, culturally responsive assessment practices. The assessment process must provide a way for persons who are homeless to identify and prioritize problems, to be engaged in a process that helps them think about and talk about their problems, and offers a way to teach goal setting and action planning.

This study sought to increase the understanding of the occupational performance problems of homeless persons and to explore the clinical utility of the COPM with this population. The specific aims of this study were to describe characteristics of homeless individuals enrolled in an occupational therapy supported employment program, and to define the self-perceived occupational performance needs of these individuals.

METHODS

Design

This descriptive study examined retrospective data generated by an occupational therapy intervention program entitled Project Employ which is located at Bethlehem Haven, a community non-profit organization serving the homeless population in Pittsburgh, Pennsylvania. Bethlehem Haven is a "one stop" homeless center that has provided both emergency shelter and transitional housing in addition to on-site supportive services to men and women experiencing homelessness for over 20 years (Bethlehem Haven, 2003). Project Employ, a grant-funded program established in 2001, is the result of a partnership between Bethlehem Haven and the occupational therapy department of Duquesne University. The program provides group and individualized support, skill-building, and intensive case management services to approximately 100 individuals each year. For a more complete description of the program, see Muñoz, Dix and Reichenbach (this volume).

Instruments

Every person enrolled in Project Employ independently completed an application to the program and participated in a screening interview with an occupational therapist to discuss their responses. Data such as the time spent homeless, and educational, vocational and criminal histories were gleaned from the application. Demographic data (age, race, ethnicity, marital status, etc.) were also collected from the screening interview. Project Employ program outcomes (enrollment status, employment outcomes, and participation in educational or volunteer activities) were acquired from Project Employ and Bethlehem Haven program databases. The *Canadian Occupational Performance Measure* (COPM) was typically completed within the first month of an applicant's enrollment. In a recent review of the psychometric properties of the COPM, Carswell and colleagues concluded that there was good evidence of test-retest reliability, discriminate, concurrent and content validity and clinical responsiveness or sensitivity to change (Carswell, McColl, Baptiste, Polatajko, & Pollack, 2004).

The COPM is designed to address the occupational therapy domains of practice (self-care, productivity, leisure) defined in the *Canadian Occupational Performance Model* (Law et al., 2005). In order to effectively explore these areas, the test manual of the COPM suggests subcategories of these domains to be used as prompts when administering the COPM. Therapists are also expected to explore additional components of these domains that arise during the interview process. As the Project Employ program has evolved, practitioners found the need to modify the subcategories used in the COPM to better address the cultural realities of persons in their program. For example, they found that the functional mobility category suggested in the self-care domain was seldom discussed. Instead, participants typically voiced issues that dealt with legal management or health and wellness problems including spirituality, and the maintenance of physical and/or mental health. Subsequently, these terms were included as sub-categories under the self-care domain. In a similar vein, paid/unpaid work and household management were useful sub-categories of the productivity domain, but the subcategory education and training was found to be more culturally relevant than school/play. Under the leisure domain, the original subcategories were maintained, but this domain was expanded to include other forms of social participation that enrollees in the program often identified as problematical, such as interactions with family, friends or within the community.

The COPM was administered as a semi-structured interview and used to engage each person in a discussion of problems in activities that they needed to, wanted to, or were expected to perform. Each identified problem was rated in terms of importance using a 1-10 scale (10 = extremely important). Each person was then asked to identify the five most important problems, which then became the focus of intervention and treatment planning. Using a similar 1-10 scale, each person rated his/her perception of performance and satisfaction with performance for each problem area. Performance and satisfaction scores were summed separately and divided by the number of problems identified which created a mean score for each.

Procedure

A retrospective review of chart data and databases maintained by Bethlehem Haven and by the Project Employ program director for every person enrolled from July 1, 2004 through June 30, 2005 (n = 97) was completed by the second author. Only data from enrollees who completed the COPM assessment (n = 65) were included in the database. Some enrollees decided they were unable to meet the expectations of the program and self-terminated, usually within the first month and prior to their completion of a COPM. Others were terminated from Project Employ to allow the participants to more effectively address a relapse in substance abuse or psychiatric illness. Data from these multiple sources were integrated into a research database created in the Statistical Package for Social Sciences (SPSS) version 11.0.1.

Data Analysis

Demographic variables were categorized and entered into a SPSS database file. In order to describe the participants in the study, descriptive statistics of these data were generated. To define the self-perceived occupational performance needs, problems identified by the participants in the COPM were coded by domain and by subcategory of these domains, and descriptive statistics of these variables were generated. Problems prioritized in the treatment planning process were analyzed in the same fashion. Narrative responses from items in the Project Employ application and verbatim goals from the COPM were entered into word processing software to support comparative analysis. These verbatim goals were analyzed using a constant comparison method (Strauss & Corbin, 1998).

RESULTS

The Participants

The majority of the participants were female (86%) and black (69%). The mean age of participants was 40.5 years with a range from 21 to 61. Approximately one-third (34%) of the participants never completed high school and a few (5%) never attended high school. Half of the enrollees (53%) had a high school diploma and of these a few (13%) had some college education. Nearly all of the applicants (92%) had participated in drug and alcohol recovery programs in the past and 83% of these were enrolled in drug treatment programs at the time of their enrollment. Over two-thirds of the respondents (68%) had received mental health services in the past and most of these (61.5%) continued to receive these services. Among those who specified a psychiatric diagnosis (n = 42), the most common diagnosis reported was depression (40%), followed by bipolar disorder (31%). Anxiety disorders were identified by 17% of these respondents and a small percentage (7%) reported being diagnosed with a psychotic disorder. Most of the applicants (88%) had criminal records.

Most enrollees (94%) were unemployed when they applied to Project Employ, but they all reported an employment history. Some had worked as recently as one month prior to enrollment, while others had not worked in over 15 years. On average, it had been nearly two years since an enrollee had been employed. Most (80%) reported having held jobs that required little to no formal training, primarily in food service, cleaning, or unskilled labor positions. The remaining participants (20%) listed jobs that likely required some amount of more formal training such as managerial and nursing assistant positions. The vast majority of the applicants who worked held low-wage positions. Some (21%) had earned salaries at or below the federal minimum wage of $5.15 and all had earned salaries that were below a living wage for the city of Pittsburgh which has been calculated at $10.39 plus benefits (Thomas Merton Center, 2005). A majority of the enrollees (74%) had some current source of regular income. Usually this was at least one form of public assistance (cash assistance, medical assistance, food stamps, SSI/SSDI).

Self-Perceived Problems

Collectively, the participants identified 612 problems. On average, participants identified 9.3 problems and rated these problems with high importance (8.84 on a 10-point scale). Just over half of these problems fell in the self-care domain (50.3%), with the other half nearly equally divided between the productivity (26.3%) and leisure (23.4%) domains. When asked to select the most pressing problems, participants prioritized 345 problems. The mean number of problems identified was 5.3. Again, participants overwhelmingly chose problems in the self-care domain (57%). Problems in the area of productivity comprised 32% of the prioritized problems, while the remaining 11% fell into the leisure domain (see Table 1).

Prioritized Problems

When applying the COPM in the treatment planning process, people are encouraged to restate the problems they have identified as most pressing into treatment goals. Each of the 345 goals identified in the COPM was categorized under one of the three primary domains of self-care, productivity and leisure. In comparative analyses, categorization proceeded using terminology grounded in the verbatim responses of the participants. Participants predominately phrased goals that were consistent with the self-care domain (59%). The most common self-care goal was "staying clean and sober," followed closely by goals for "obtaining housing" or "improving physical or mental health." Other types of self-care goals

TABLE 1. Distribution of COPM Problems

Total Problems Identified N = 612		% of Domain	% of Total Problems	Prioritized Problems Identified N = 345		% of Domain	% of Total Problems
Self-Care Domain	*308*		*50.3*	*Self-Care Domain*	*196*		*56.8%*
Personal Care	9	2.9	1.5	Personal Care	2	1.0	.06%
Health and Wellness	142	46.1	23.2	Health and Wellness	101	51.5	29.2%
Legal Management	57	18.5	9.3	Legal Management	30	15.3	8.7%
Community Mgmt	100	32.5	16.3	Community Mgmt	63	32.1	18.2%
Productivity Domain	*161*		*26.3*	*Productivity Domain*	*112*		*32.5%*
Program	10.6	10.6	1.7	Program	10	8.9	3.0%
Paid/Unpaid Work	71	44.1	11.6	Paid/Unpaid Work	52	46.4	15.1%
Home	8	5.0	1.3	Home	3	2.6	.87%
Education	65	40.4	10.6	Education	47	41.9	16.6%
Leisure Domain	*143*		*23.4*	*Leisure Domain*	*37*		*10.7%*
Quiet Leisure	23	16.1	3.0	Quiet Leisure	5	13.5	1.4%
Active Leisure	33	23.1	5.4	Active Leisure	7	18.9	2.0%
Social Leisure	20	14.0	3.3	Social Leisure	5	13.5	1.4%
Family Interaction	33	23.1	5.4	Family Interaction	14	37.8	4.0%
Friend Interaction	17	11.9	2.8	Friend Interaction	4	10.8	1.2%
Community Interaction	17	11.9	2.8	Community Interaction	2	5.4	.06%

included learning budgeting skills or meeting probation requirements. Almost one-third (31%) of the verbatim goals could be classified as being in the productivity domain. Here the most prominent goal was to obtain either part or full-time employment. Other very common goals included the pursuit of an education or GED certification, or to start a volunteer position. Only a few of the goals (10%) could be categorized as fitting in the leisure domain. In this domain, participants were most likely to define a goal to improve the quality of interpersonal relationships, especially with family members, while goals for increasing leisure pursuits were far less common (See Table 2). Table 3 compares the distribution of occupational performance problems reported by this population of homeless individuals with populations in previous studies. In general, the participants in this study identified a higher percentage of problems in the self-care and productivity domains and a lower percentage of problems in the leisure domain than previous studies (Chesworth et al., 2002; Pan et al., 2003; Tryssenaar et al., 1999).

TABLE 2. Categorization of Verbatim COPM Goals

Verbatim Goals	Number of Goals	Percentage of Domain
Self Care Domain 205/345–59% of all goals		
Stay Clean	43	21%
Obtain Permanent Housing	37	18%
Increase Physical Health	31	15%
Legal Assistance; Meet Probation; Pay Fines	30	15%
Maintain Mental Health	22	11%
Increase Budgeting	14	7%
Improve ADL/Life Skills	10	5%
Increase Spiritual Health	9	4%
Get Transportation	9	4%
Productivity Domain 107/345–31% of all goals		
Obtain PT/FT Employment	41	38%
Pursue Education/Go Back to School	30	28%
Start Volunteer Work	17	16%
Gain Computer Skills	16	15%
Enroll in/Complete Project Employ Courses	3	3%
Leisure Domain 34/345–10% of all goals		
Increase Quality of Interpersonal Relationships	24	71%
Improve Quiet Time/Quiet Recreation	10	29%

TABLE 3. Distribution of Identified Problems: A Comparison

Study	Population	Self-Care	Productivity	Leisure
Current Study	Homeless Individuals (N = 65)	59%	31%	10%
Tryssenaar et al. (1999)	Homeless Individuals (N = 25)	48%	27%	25%
Pan et al. (2003)	Taiwanese MH Disability (N = 141)	37%*	25%*	20%*
Chesworth et al. (2002)	British MH Disability (N = 60)	15.3%	22.5%	62.2%
McColl et al. (2000)	Community dwelling individuals with physical disabilities (N = 61)	45.6%	23%	31.4%

**Note:* Pan et al. (2003) categorized identified problems into 5 areas: self care (37%), leisure (25%), productivity (20%), social encounters (12%) and other (6%).

DISCUSSION

The findings reported in this study indicate that the COPM facilitated person-centered, culturally responsive assessment with homeless individuals. For the therapist, the assessment provided a means to engage participants in a structured process of problem identification. The conversational format of the assessment process seemed to engage participants in an interpersonal process where discussion of potentially uncomfortable topics could be effectively addressed. The use of the COPM in occupational therapy programs serving homeless populations has not been well documented. Tryssenaar et al. (1999) reported that the COPM supported person-centered assessment with homeless individuals in an emergency shelter. The present study differs in several ways. In Tryssenaar's study, there was no occupational therapy programming occurring at the shelter and the data were collected by students over a five-day period. In the present study, data were collected at a homeless center offering residential care for persons enrolled in an occupational therapy-supported employment program. The clinicians who collected the data usually employed the COPM within a month of a person's enrollment which offered them time to develop a relationship and some level of rapport with each person.

Given the complex set of problems a person who is homeless can bring to the clinical encounter and the fact that the homeless are such a heterogeneous population, it is encouraging that the COPM supported the identification and prioritization of problems. Demographic data collected in this study reflected a population who were not only homeless, but also usually poor, with limited vocational histories, mental health disabilities, and addictions. Use of the COPM helped generate a description of the self-perceived occupational performance problems specific to this population. Modifications to subcategories of the COPM domains seemed to address critical issues in the participants' lives as reflected in the number of problems identified in content subcategories that were added to the COPM (e.g., legal management, housing, education and training, etc.).

The distribution of problems identified in the three domain areas differed from the distribution of problems identified with other homeless populations (Tryssenaar et al., 1999), and from studies of individuals with mental health disabilities (Chesworth et al., 2002; Pan et al., 2003). In general, this population identified a higher percentage of their problems in the self-care and productivity domains and a far lower percentage of their problems in the leisure domain. Modification of the subcategories may have influenced the participants' identification of occupational performance problems which in turn may have influenced the types of goals that were selected. However, since the subcategories that were added were grounded in trends of problem identification that had been established by using the COPM with this population for over two years, the researchers are confident that the distribution reflects a culturally responsive assessment process.

It should be noted that the practitioners used the subcategories only as an opening to discuss potential problems and did not offer a predetermined set of problem or goal areas which could have led the participants to respond in particular ways (Candler, 2003). It is more likely that the structure and expected outcomes of the on-site residential programs that many of the participants came from and the focus on the development of productive time use by the occupational therapy program had a stronger effect on the distribution of identified problems. Participants may have internalized programmatic expectations that emphasized continued efforts towards recovery and expectations for the development of productive occupational roles. On the other hand, while these external influences may have influenced a person's identification of problems, program expectations were felt to be less likely to influence a person's internal perspective of the importance of their goals. The mean importance rating was quite high (8.84 on a 10-point scale).

Self-Perceived Problems of Self-Care

Most of the problems identified by participants fell in the self-care domain. While other studies have demonstrated a similar finding (see Table 3), the themes defined in qualitative analysis of verbatim goals provide insight into how self-care may be perceived by homeless populations. In previous studies, the self-care problems identified by individuals with physical disabilities often included basic ADLs such as dressing, transfers, and hygiene (Chan & Lee, 1997; Chen et al., 2003). In this study, the most frequent self-care problems were maintaining sobriety and/or staying drug free, obtaining housing, managing legal problems, and maintaining physical or mental health. The prevalence of drug or alcohol addiction (Steinhaus et al., 2004) and mental illness (Jones et al., 2003) is a well-established finding in studies of the homeless. The fact that the participants in this study prioritized issues of mental health and addiction treatment could reflect some level of insight into these problems; however, this emphasis could also have been influenced by the presence of onsite drug and alcohol programs. In addition, sobriety is a requirement of enrollment into Project Employ and many of the residential programs where these participants have found housing.

Self-Perceived Problems of Productivity

Approximately one-third of the problems (31%) identified by participants were in the productivity domain. This finding is comparable with other studies which have found problems in this domain accounting for anywhere from 22.5% (Chesworth et al., 2002) to 27% of all identified problems (Tryssenaar et al., 1999). This finding is not unexpected in a program that supports the development of worker, student and volunteer roles. Project Employ practitioners who administered the COPM reported that participants who do not spontaneously identify problems and develop goals related to these types of productive activities are often encouraged to explore a productive role to pursue. Nonetheless, despite the vocational nature of the program, these participants identified nearly twice as many goals in the self-care domain. It is possible that these participants' prioritization of self-care over productivity reflects a need to acquire some personal stability before engaging in functional roles.

Self-Perceived Problems of Leisure

Only 10% of the identified problems were categorized in the leisure domain. Most other studies have reported that problems in this domain account for between 20% (Law et al., 1994; Pan et al., 2003) to 62% (Chesworth et al., 2002) of all problems. The unique distribution in this population may have multiple explanations. It is possible that participants have little experience pursuing avocational interests and the subcategories of active, quiet, and social leisure may lack cultural relevance. Alternatively, Project Employ participants may be so focused on attaining a productive role, or housing and health issues, that they do not feel that it is appropriate to have goals related to leisure pursuits. In addition, many participants live in residential settings with program requirements that keep them engaged for most of the day. These requirements may restrict time for leisure activities. Finally, the location of the leisure section on the actual assessment may influence problem identification in this area. A majority of goals identified by participants in this study were in the self-care and productivity domains. By the time the discussion turns to leisure, a participant may feel that they have already identified an adequate number of problems in the assessment process.

Limitations of the Study

The primary limitation of this study is that the findings are specific to the setting. This study reports the results of initial COPM assessments for 65 participants at an urban homeless center in downtown Pittsburgh, Pennsylvania. This setting may have influenced the demographics of the participants and the difficulties they experienced. For example, chronically homeless populations are less likely to make contact with helping organizations (Kuhn & Culhane, 1998) and more likely to have a co-morbid mental health disability and addiction (Phelan & Link, 1999). Participants in this study were enrolled in a grant-funded occupational therapy program that emphasized employment, education and volunteerism as primary outcomes. Homeless populations in programs that do not emphasize these outcomes may identify other patterns of occupational performance problems.

Implications for Practice

The results of this study suggest implications for both assessment and intervention strategies for practitioners working with homeless populations in community settings. Practitioners are encouraged to take advantage of the flexibility inherent in the administration of the COPM. This tool offers practitioners an effective method for integrating assessment and treatment planning in an efficient, person-centered process. Minor modifications to subcategories of the domains of occupational performance defined in the COPM can support an assessment process that is more consistent with the cultural realities of homeless individuals without jeopardizing the integrity of the COPM or the *Canadian Occupational Performance Model* on which it is based. Knowledge of the types of occupational performance problems identified by persons who are homeless may assist practitioners to ask more culturally responsive questions and elicit more accurate identification of the person's problems. Finally, the pattern of performance problems defined in this population suggests that while community programs may have their own expectations for program outcomes, practitioners must recognize and may need to prioritize the person's basic self-care needs before addressing limitations in productive roles such as student, worker or volunteer. A person-centered, culturally responsive assessment process can facilitate the use of occupational therapy interventions which are both meaningful and relevant.

REFERENCES

Bethlehem Haven (2003). *Welcome to the haven.* Retrieved September 5, 2005, from http://www.bethlehemhaven.org/

Candler, C. (2003). Sensory integration and therapeutic riding at summer camp: Occupational performance outcomes. *Physical & Occupational Therapy in Pediatrics, 23*, 3, 51-65.

Carswell, A., McColl, M., Baptiste, S. M., Polatajko, H., & Pollock, N. (2004). The Canadian Occupational Performance Measure: A research and clinical literature review. *Canadian Journal of Occupational Therapy, 71*, 210-222.

Chan, C. & Lee, T. (1997). Validity of the Canadian Occupational Performance Measure. *Occupational Therapy International, 4*, 229-47.

Chesworth, C., Duffy, R., Hodnett, J., & Knight, A. (2002). Measuring clinical effectiveness in mental health: Is the Canadian Occupational Performance an appropriate measure? *British Journal of Occupational Therapy, 65*, 30-36.

Finlayson, M., Baker, M., Rodman, L., & Herzberg, G. (2002). The process and outcomes of a multimethod needs assessment at a homeless shelter. *American Journal of Occupational Therapy, 56*, 313-321.

Gonzalez, G. & Rosenheck, R.A. (2002). Outcomes and service use among homeless persons with serious mental illness and substance abuse. *Psychiatric Services, 53*, 437-446.

Hwang, S.W. (2001). Homelessness and health. *Canadian Medical Association Journal, 164*, 229-233.

Jones, K., Colson, P.W., Holter, M.C., Lin, S., Valencia, J.D., Susser, E., & Wyatt, R.J. (2003). Cost-effectiveness of critical time intervention to reduce homelessness among persons with mental illness. *Psychiatric Services, 54*, 884-890.

Kronenberg, F., Algado, S.S., & Pollard, N. (2005). *Occupational therapy without borders: Learning from the spirit of survivors.* Edinburgh: Elsevier Churchill Livingstone.

Kuhn, R. & Culhane, D.P. (1998). Applying cluster analysis to test a typology of homelessness by pattern of shelter utilization: Results from the analysis of administrative data. *American Journal of Community Psychology, 26*, 207-232.

Law, M., Baptiste, S., Carswell, A., McColl, M.A., Polatajko, H., & Pollock, N. (2005). *Canadian Occupational Performance Measure, 4th edition*. Ottawa: Canadian Association of Occupational Therapists, Inc.

Law, M., Polatajko, H., Pollock, N., McColl, M.A., Carswell, A., & Baptiste, S. (1994). The Canadian Occupational Performance Measure: Results of pilot testing. *Canadian Journal of Occupational Therapy, 61*, 191-197.

McColl, M.A., Patterson, M., Davies, D., Doubt, L., & Law, M. (2000). Validity and community utility of the Canadian Occupational Performance Measure. *Canadian Journal of Occupational Therapy, 67*, 22-30.

Muñoz, J.P., Reichenbach, D., & Hansen, A.M. (2005). Project Employ: Engineering hope and breaking down barriers in homelessness. *WORK: A Journal of Prevention, Assessment, and Rehabilitation, 25*, 241-252.

Muñoz, J., Dix, S. & Reichenbach, D. (this volume). Building productive roles: Occupational therapy in a homeless shelter. *Occupational Therapy in Health Care.*

O'Toole, S.M., & Withers, J.S. (1998). From the streets, to the emergency department and back: A model of emergency care for the homeless. *Emergency Medicine, 20*, 12-20.

Pan, A., Chung, L., & Hsin-Hwei, G. (2003). Reliability and validity of the Canadian Occupational Performance Measure for clients with psychiatric disorders in Taiwan. *Occupational Therapy International, 10*, 269-277.

Steinhaus, D.A., Harley, D.A., & Rogers, J. (2004). Homelessness and people with affective disorders and other mental illness. *Journal of Applied Rehabilitation Counseling, 35*, 36-40.

Strauss, A. & Corbin, J. (1998). *Basics of qualitative research: Techniques and procedures for developing grounded theory*. Thousand Oaks: Sage Publications.

Thomas Merton Center. *What is a living wage in Allegheny County?* Accessed September 12, 2005, from http://www.thomasmertoncenter.org/laborpledge/moreinfo.htm

Tryssenaar, J., Jones, E.J., & Lee, D. (1999). Occupational performance needs of a shelter population. *Canadian Journal of Occupational Therapy, 66*, 188-195.

doi:10.1300/J003v20n03_09

Occupational Therapy Intervention to Foster Goal Setting Skills for Homeless Mothers

Winifred Schultz-Krohn, PhD, OTR/L, BCP, SWC, FAOTA
Skye Drnek, BS, OTI
Kelly Powell, BS, OTI

SUMMARY. Occupational therapy intervention was provided to two mothers living in a homeless shelter to foster goal setting skills and the ability to develop a systematic method to meet those goals. The Model of Human Occupation (MOHO) was used as the theoretical framework to guide intervention. Both mothers were able to establish personal goals and work towards meeting those goals but the outcomes varied. The difference in outcomes between the two mothers is described using MOHO with analysis of how occupational therapy services can be used with homeless mothers. doi:10.1300/J003v20n03_10 *[Article copies available for a fee from The Haworth Document Delivery Service: 1-800-HAWORTH. E-mail address: <docdelivery@haworthpress.com> Website: <http://www.HaworthPress.com> © 2006 by The Haworth Press, Inc. All rights reserved.]*

Winifred Schultz-Krohn, Skye Drnek, and Kelly Powell are all affiliated with the Department of Occupational Therapy, San Jose State University.

Address correspondence to: Winifred Schultz-Krohn, Department of Occupational Therapy, San Jose State University, One Washington Square, San Jose, CA 95192-0059 (E-mail: winifred@casa.sjsu.edu)

[Haworth co-indexing entry note]: "Occupational Therapy Intervention to Foster Goal Setting Skills for Homeless Mothers." Schultz-Krohn, Winifred, Skye Drnek, and Kelly Powell. Co-published simultaneously in *Occupational Therapy in Health Care* (The Haworth Press, Inc.) Vol. 20, No. 3/4, 2006, pp. 149-166; and: *Homelessness in America: Perspectives, Characterizations, and Considerations for Occupational Therapy* (ed: Kathleen Swenson Miller, Georgiana L. Herzberg, and Sharon A. Ray) The Haworth Press, Inc., 2006, pp. 149-166. Single or multiple copies of this article are available for a fee from The Haworth Document Delivery Service [1-800-HAWORTH, 9:00 a.m. - 5:00 p.m. (EST). E-mail address: docdelivery@haworthpress.com].

Available online at http://othc.haworthpress.com
© 2006 by The Haworth Press, Inc. All rights reserved.
doi:10.1300/J003v20n03_10

KEYWORDS. Occupational therapy, homeless mothers, goal setting skills, Model of Human Occupation

LITERATURE REVIEW

Homelessness is defined as a lack of "a fixed, regular, and adequate nighttime residence" (National Coalition for the Homeless, 2004). Homelessness can be viewed as a point-in-time problem where a family is homeless on a specific day but recent investigations demonstrate that the majority of the homeless population experiences marginal housing for an extended time. The longitudinal pattern of homelessness most often includes alternating periods of being housed and homeless within a year (National Coalition for the Homeless, 2004). Approximately 1%, or 3.5 million, of the U.S. population experiences homelessness each year; approximately 38% of them are children (Urban Institute, 2000). Families are the fastest growing portion of the homeless population and currently constitute 41% of the total homeless population within the United States (Turner, 2004; U.S. Conference of Mayors, 2003). The configuration of homeless families is most often a mother with two to three dependent children (Bassuk, Browne, & Buckner, 1996).

There is substantial literature describing the characteristics and experiences of homeless families (Banyard & Graham-Bermann, 1995; Bassuk et al., 1996; Baumann, 1993; Choi & Snyder, 1999; Hausman & Hammen, 1993; MacKnee & Mervyn, 2002; Menke & Wagner, 1997; Thrasher & Mowbray, 1995). Literature documents increased stress and depression, the deterioration of parental roles, and a loss of social supports for mothers who are homeless. Davis and Kutter (1998), working with homeless women, identified specific deficits in occupational performance, such as financial management. Although investigations have provided rich descriptions of the experience of homeless families, there has been little research that focuses on effective intervention strategies to foster occupational performance in homeless mothers (Lindsey, 2000). Several authors have recommended that occupational therapy services should be provided for the homeless population and suggestions have been made for various forms of intervention (Davis & Kutter, 1998; Heubner & Tryssenaar, 1996; Kearney, 1991; Schultz-Krohn, 2004; Townsend & Wilcock, 2004; Tryssenaar, Jones, & Lee, 1999). These services have not been fully implemented and the limited literature that exists describes the results of occupational therapy intervention with children (Drake, 1992) and single women (Kavanagh & Fares, 1995). The homeless population remains underserved by occupational therapy.

Hausman and Hammen argue that "the shelter experience offers a rare opportunity to provide clear and direct assistance within the context of nurturance and support" (1993, p. 366). Occupational therapy is uniquely equipped to provide intervention in a shelter environment by blending the concepts of occupation, enabling, and justice to meet the needs of this population (Townsend & Wilcock, 2004). All three of these interrelated concepts are applicable to homeless mothers and, when used in best practice, will support occupational performance and roles. Using a solution-focused and strength-based approach has been advocated when working with homeless mothers (Lindsey, 2000). This case study investigation describes occupational therapy intervention provided for two homeless mothers living in a family shelter. The intervention focused on helping these two mothers create realistic and systematic goals that were solution-focused and led to positive outcomes.

METHOD

A case study methodology was used in this investigation. Case study methods can effectively be used to understand the unique features of an individual or to provide insight into a specific situation (Stake, 1994; Yin, 2003). The most vital aspect of a case study design is the investigation of a single phenomenon; the phenomenon may include one or several individuals (Depoy & Gitlin, 1998). A case study has also been described as an effective method for addressing "a relatively short, self-contained episode or segment of a person's life" (Bromley, 1989, p. 1). Bromley (1989) identifies several basic rules for designing and conducting a case study that include providing a statement of a clear objective and an ecological context for the case. This investigation was directed towards understanding the importance of creating meaningful goals with mothers living in a temporary homeless shelter exclusively for families. The process of creating the goals included intervention to develop the skills necessary to meet the goal and convert the skills into habits to support occupational performance (Rogers, 2000). In this manner goals were not abstract but were solution-focused and the two mothers provided ongoing assessment of the importance of their goals (Lindsey, 2000).

The occupational therapy services were provided by two graduate occupational therapy interns completing their Fieldwork Level II experience. The interns were supervised by an experienced clinician who developed and supervised the intern program at this shelter for six years. This investigation was limited to the length of fieldwork experience, three months.

Setting

This investigation occurred at an emergency homeless shelter in a Northern California county. The shelter is specifically designed for homeless families and defines a family as an adult over the age of 18 who is responsible for a child under the age of 18. Configurations have included grandparents caring for grandchildren, mothers and dependent children, fathers and dependent children, and two-parent families, although most homeless families residing at this shelter are mothers with dependent children.

The physical environment of the shelter allows a degree of privacy and provides families with a separate 12 foot-by-12 foot room. Families use a communal bathroom. Three meals a day are provided for all residing at the shelter. The shelter does have specific rules and requirements that must be followed to remain at the shelter. These include no drug or alcohol use, evidence of an active job and housing search, and the completion of chores at the shelter. This a temporary supportive housing shelter where families can remain for up to three months.

Although the shelter assigns a case manager to each family residing at the shelter, the case manager does not establish systematic goals with families. The case manager is responsible for monitoring family compliance with the shelter rules, providing suggestions regarding resources, and meeting with the family two to three times a month to monitor progress in securing housing. No occupational therapy services are offered on a consistent basis at the shelter. For the past six summers, an experienced occupational therapist has implemented and supervised an occupational therapy Fieldwork Level II program to provide services to the shelter. Services are provided to people residing at the shelter on both a group and an individual basis to foster and support occupational performance. The shelter actively seeks these services on an ongoing basis and respects the occupational therapy services provided by the interns and supervisor.

Measures

The Occupational Self Assessment (OSA Version 2.1) was administered during the initial occupational therapy session (Baron, Kielhofner, Iyneger, Goldhammer, & Wolenski, 2002). This tool is based on the model of human occupation (MOHO) and serves as a client-centered method of data collection (Kielhofner, 2002). This assessment was selected because it supports client goal development and is relatively quick to administer. Homeless parents often face many constraints on their time and selecting an instrument that can be completed in approximately 30 minutes was a criteria. The OSA provides specific statements related to occupational performance and the client rates both perceived competence in performance and the level of importance to the individual, using a four-point scale. The OSA supports and guides the client in developing goals by selecting areas of occupational performance identified as important to the client. The OSA also fosters the therapeutic relationship between the therapist and client through the collaborative assessment process.

The Beck Depression Inventory -II (BDI -II) was also administered to both women by the third occupational therapy session (Beck, Steer, & Brown, 1996). The BDI is a self-assessment tool consisting of 21 groups of statements that help determine a client's possible level of depression. This measure was included to provide additional information about both mothers that would direct intervention services.

Data Collection

Detailed progress notes were completed following each session which identified the focus of the session and the relationship of the services to the client's stated goals. Included in the notes were both subjective and objective information provided by each mother. Each mother was asked to assess the effectiveness of the session and provide additional information regarding her respective goals.

Analysis of Data

Data collected throughout the course of intervention was analyzed using a constant comparative method whereby subsequent sessions were compared to previous sessions to search for change and relationships (Landry, 2001). This process involved in-depth discussions between the two graduate interns and the supervising therapist. The theoretical framework that guided intervention was MOHO and the data collected was compared to this model for interpretation.

The model of human occupation provided a framework to understand the complexities of roles and habits (Kielhofner, 2002). Roles are supported by both internal constructs and external environmental features. For many parents, the experience of being homeless represents a conflict between an internally endorsed role and the external environment (Banyard & Graham-Bermann, 1995; Menke & Wagner, 1997). The internalized role of being a parent includes the responsibility of child care. The shelter environment often diminishes parental authority and control by positioning parents in a subordinate role to shelter workers where decisions about a child's behavior, meals, and bathing routines are dictated by someone other than the parent (Schultz-Krohn, 2004). Previously established habits and routines that supported the parental role are often markedly altered when residing in a homeless shelter (Baumann, 1993). The ability to establish and work towards achieving self-identified goals was seen as a means to support parental roles. This reflects the constructs of volition including personal causation and occupational choice articulated by MOHO.

Trustworthiness of analysis and results was addressed through several means (Krefting, 1991). Both interns engaged in reflective dialogue with the supervisor several times a week to examine how data was interpreted. Interpretation was also shared at meetings with the respective case managers to gain an additional perspective. Case managers not only concurred with the interpretation but praised the efforts on the intervention program in helping each mother begin the process of setting a goal. Triangulation of data was also accomplished through discussions with each mother individually regarding the meaning of the goals established and the process of systematically reaching those goals. Although both mothers lived at the shelter during the same time period, no data was shared between mothers in order to maintain confidentiality.

Participants

Two mothers were included in the case study investigation. Both were referred for occupational therapy services from their respective case managers at the shelter because they had not made progress in developing and implementing personal goals that would extricate them from homelessness. Both mothers agreed to participate in intervention services and signed consent was secured prior to the evaluation session. Consent meant that data would be shared with respective case managers but not between each mother. The history shared during the occupational therapy sessions is provided as a temporal context for each mother.

Amy's History

Amy was a 36-year-old Caucasian woman who was referred to occupational therapy services for work readiness. She reported having significant learning disabilities and had experienced head trauma due to parental abuse and domestic violence. Amy was chronically abused by her mother from the ages of 1 1/2 -14 years old and was placed in foster care during adolescence. As an adult, a previous male partner abused her several times a week over the course of four years. She had severe depression as identified from the results of the BDI-II. She stated that she has both long-term and short-term memory loss. At the time of this investigation she lived with her partner of 6 years who fathered two of her six children, ranging in ages from 17 months-15 years. One child passed away at 3 months old. At the time, Amy had custody of her youngest child, while her oldest daughter lived with her mother and the whereabouts of her other children were unknown. Amy and her partner were currently taking the steps needed to regain custody of their other child. Amy completed the 10th grade of school, but did not receive her diploma. She dropped out of school in the 11th grade when she became pregnant with her first child.

Carrie's History

Carrie was a 23-year-old Hispanic woman who was referred to occupational therapy services for pain management due to back and neck pain, work readiness, and financial management skills. She completed high school and had completed some vocational training. She had moderate to severe depression as identified by the BDI-II. Carrie gave birth to a 4 week premature son before coming to the shelter. Her son was 7 weeks old when she began receiving occupational therapy services. She believed that her current partner was the child's father but was unable to confirm this belief. She had not pursued paternity testing. Her current partner did not live with her at the shelter and was living in his boss's residence. He was employed but did not have a steady job and was financially unstable. Carrie grew up in an unstable home with an alcoholic mother. She maintained weekly contact with her sister and monthly contact with her parents but she sought to live at the shelter with her newborn son. She appeared overwhelmed by the birth of her son, her new living situation in the homeless shelter, her family life, and the relationship with her boyfriend.

INTERVENTION

Intervention was provided on an individual basis approximately two times per week for a two-month period. Sessions were generally between 30 and 45 minutes in length and were scheduled at times convenient for each mother. Sessions were designed to address the specific goals identified by each mother using a basic structure of discussing the goal, identifying the techniques to meet the goal, engaging in the techniques, developing a plan for working on the goal until the next session, evaluating the effectiveness of the session, and identifying the focus of the next session. Developing systematic goals with a clear outcome was an important feature of the intervention services provided. This method allowed each mother to establish a clear goal and identify when the goal was accomplished, thereby endorsing a sense of personal choice and efficacy. The techniques to meet the established goals varied as can be seen in the description below.

Amy's Goals

It was apparent during the initial meeting with Amy that she was extremely willing to share information to develop an intervention plan. She rated 17 of the possible 20 occupational performance items on the OSA as being most important in her life, with the remaining 3 items considered as more important. From this information, it was interpreted that Amy had difficulty in prioritizing items of importance in her life. The structure of the OSA, with support from the intern, allowed Amy to systematically choose four areas in her life she wanted to improve. With the occupational therapy intern, she created three goals addressing time management, financial management, and interview skills. She had a job interview later that same day which allowed the intern and Amy to discuss strategies necessary for a successful interview. Amy was unprepared to answer questions about her previous employment history and had not considered her personal appearance as a factor during the interview. These issues were specifically addressed during the initial session with Amy. This reflects the ability of the intervention to focus on immediate needs and collaborate on solution-focused strategies to meet her goal of becoming employed.

It was found that a core issue surrounding many of Amy's concerns was her inability to manage her time effectively. This was addressed by first discussing options and then jointly selecting a method. A weekly planner was introduced and support was provided to help Amy record upcoming appointments. After attempting to use the planner for two days, Amy reported confusion at the complexity of the planner. It needed to be simplified by breaking it into half-hour segments during the day. Amy then understood how to enter her schedule into the planner and meet her goal of arriving to appointments on time. At each subsequent occupational therapy session, Amy was asked how the planner was working and if she needed any further assistance to use this device. Amy was able to provide feedback on the effectiveness of the planner and the importance of time management in her daily life. The intern provided reinforcement for the use of this device. This exchange also sought to convert the skills of time management into a habit in Amy's daily life. Time management was also addressed as Amy arrived for each occupational therapy session. Amy was complimented when she arrived on time and received encouragement to arrive on time for the following appointment. When Amy arrived late for an appointment, a few moments were taken to discuss factors that impeded Amy's time management skills.

After six weeks of intervention, Amy demonstrated self-initiative to request help in areas of perceived weakness including budgeting and financial management skills. She was unable to balance a check book and had significant difficulties establishing a monthly budget. Amy was provided with various materials to develop a budget with her partner. This intervention was designed not only to increase math and budgeting skills but also to provide an opportunity to practice communication skills, previously learned in an occupational therapy group session, with her partner. It became apparent to Amy that they would not be successful in completing the materials and Amy asked to develop the necessary skills to plan a budget during the next intervention session. This serves as an example of Amy's ability to identify a goal and seek the resources necessary to reach the goal. Although developing the skills needed to meet the budgeting goal took longer than anticipated, Amy was able to achieve all three goals set during the initial evaluation. She received a total of 12 individual sessions.

Throughout the course of intervention Amy identified other goals she wanted to address during occupational therapy intervention, including her role as a mother. Amy and her case manager had both expressed concerns over Amy's diminished verbal interaction with her young son. Concerns were also identified regarding Amy's inconsistencies with discipline. Amy felt poorly equipped to effectively reinforce the behaviors she wanted to support in her son. To achieve this goal, intervention focused on the acquisition of tools Amy could use when interacting with her son.

Amy did not have positive parental role models as a child and that lack of a model may have contributed to her parenting difficulties (Hausman & Hammen, 1993). Again, the process of clearly identifying the goal, selecting the necessary skills to be developed, and practicing those skills to foster habit formation was used. Amy was taught to communicate with her son using simple words and baby signs, what the role of mother encompasses, play and interaction techniques, and community resources available for mothers. Individual intervention was also provided for her son. The Denver Developmental Screening Test-II (DDST-II) was administered and it identified possible developmental concerns in the areas of personal-social, fine motor-adaptive, and language (Frankenburg, Dodds, Archer, Shapiro, & Bresnick, 1992). The focus of intervention for Amy's son was fostering skills that would enable Amy to experience reciprocity in their relationship including communication, eye contact, task completion, clean-up skills, and following directions. At the time of discharge, Amy had been living in permanent housing for approximately one week, had been hired for her dream job as cashier at a local store, and had registered to begin taking classes at the local community college to pursue her graduate equivalency degree (G.E.D.) as well as take other classes to pursue restaurant management.

Carrie's Goals

Carrie was able to rate her level of competence, or her ability in specific areas of occupational performance, and the value she placed on the items using the OSA. However, she did rate 10 of 20 items as being most important to her in her life. Similar to Amy, this was interpreted as a difficulty in prioritizing occupational performance. From the OSA and initial interview, it appeared that Carrie had low self-confidence and she undervalued her skills. She had difficulty accepting compliments and validating her occupation as mother. She created three goals addressing time management skills, resuming a dance routine to address her weight gain during pregnancy, and pain management to reduce her back pain. Although moving from the shelter was also identified as important, Carrie did not want to address that goal during the initial occupational therapy sessions.

Carrie appeared very honest with her answers and concerns; she stated that she had no interest in obtaining a job or going to classes, but that she wanted to focus on caring for her son. The first topic addressed with Carrie was her pain and physical limitations that impacted her ability to hold and care for her son. Carrie was receptive to suggestions and strategies to improve body mechanics, however, it did not appear that she would continue these exercises independently. She required ongoing support and encouragement to practice appropriate body mechanics to decrease back pain. These skills did not readily convert to habits within her daily routine of caring for her son.

It also became apparent after only a few intervention sessions that Carrie's boyfriend was a significant factor influencing her ability to meet her goal of achieving independent living. Carrie would immediately abandon any appointments or meetings if he called and wanted to see her. She did not have plans to live with him, but her interactions with him were a priority that prevented her from accomplishing her stated goals.

Although Carrie had identified that she did not have an interest in obtaining a job, she focused on updating her resume during the first few intervention sessions. It appeared that Carrie needed a concrete goal to accomplish. It also became apparent that Carrie had many ideas about what she wanted in life, however, no idea how to accomplish her goals. She appeared frustrated with herself and her situation, with no method of extricating herself from being homeless. In the following intervention sessions, Carrie did complete her resume and appeared satisfied that she had completed one goal even though it was not a goal established at the beginning of the intervention.

Carrie often expressed that she felt unable to succeed in her role as parent. She stated that she felt her interaction skills were limited and her relationship with her son had deteriorated. This became the primary goal of subsequent intervention sessions. Carrie was concerned that her pain was prohibiting her interactions with her son and that this would negatively impact his overall development. The therapist suggested administering the DDST-II to her son. She appeared very excited when her son passed all items for his developmental age. During Carrie's interaction with her son, she smiled each time she was praised for her ability to parent. This praise also served to reinforce her role as mother. The importance of incorporating her son into all of Carrie's goals and future intervention sessions was apparent; incorporating her son was very meaningful and worthwhile to Carrie and would allow Carrie to achieve the greatest amount of success in her goals.

To address her role as mother as well as her back pain, Carrie learned to use proper body mechanics incorporated into her daily interactions with her son. She practiced them at each successive intervention session and was reminded about the importance of making them a habit. By using pillows to prop herself up and applying the principles of proper body mechanics, Carrie was also taught how to position her son in her lap in order to interact with him as well as read to him. She said that reading was positive for her as well because she had decreased confidence in her ability to read. Increasing her reading skills would help her in future employment. Each successive intervention session continued to address the most important role to Carrie, her role of mother, as well as planning for a job and permanent housing. She stated that she could not take big leaps all at once, but that she was slowly making goals and accomplishing things. Time management was also addressed by discussing its importance to Carrie, the importance of having a routine for herself and her son, and by introducing a daily planner. Carrie did not continue to use a day planner; however, she began to carry a notebook with her to keep reminders in for herself as well as questions and concerns to ask other professionals during meetings. During the last two weeks of intervention, it appeared that Carrie's anxiety over her limited time to remain at the shelter was increasing. She appeared extremely frustrated with her body, as if saying, "I hate my body, my body is not working the way I want it to right now, this is keeping me from accomplishing my goals." Intervention again addressed her body mechanics through simple exercises and Carrie experienced some pain relief, however, was unable to make the exercises a habit.

At termination of the intervention services, Carrie was still living at the shelter, had no job or educational prospects, and had no definite housing secured when her time at the shelter was terminated. She had one possible housing prospect that included rent reduction in exchange for help managing the property but stated that it would not work because her boyfriend was not willing to move in with her and help support her and her son. She did acknowledge that she had improved in parenting skills but was concerned that she was unable to provide housing for herself and her son.

RESULTS

Intervention services provided for both mothers had facilitated positive changes in their respective lives. Through the course of intervention a trusting relationship was developed with the therapist because the mothers' opinions were validated and they could work on their personal goals. Validation, or respecting the client's perspective and experience, is stated as being necessary for effective therapy and played a role in the intervention results (Kielhofner & Forsyth, 2002). In the past, other professionals had ignored Carrie's concerns about her back pain, however, her therapist validated her concern by incorporating pain management and proper body mechanics into her intervention program. From that point forward,

Carrie expressed that she appreciated that the occupational therapy intern took into account her voice and concerns.

Volition

Throughout the intervention process, there were marked similarities and differences between Amy and Carrie. The most profound difference was that of volition, which is seen as one's sense of self-efficacy along with one's values, interests, and beliefs (Kielhofner, 2002; Kavanagh & Fares, 1995). The construct of volition includes that of personal causation where a person acknowledges a "sense of competence and effectiveness" (Kielhofner, 2002, p. 15). Both mothers initially reported a diminished ability to achieve desired goals. During the first session clear goals were collaboratively developed with a specific targeted outcome. Strategies to meet the goal were discussed and decided upon in a joint problem-solving manner. The ability to establish systematic goals with a strategy to achieve the goals served as a foundation for the intervention provided.

Amy seemed to know what was needed of her in order to establish and meet her goals but did not have the strategies needed to get there. Many homeless women have the desire to change their lives but do not have the tools to bring about these positive changes (Menke & Wagner, 1997). When occupational therapy services began, Amy was actively seeking employment but did not have the skills needed for successful interviewing, such as considering appropriate appearance, the importance of punctuality, and how to answer critical questions about past work history. Through the intervention services Amy developed a sense of security and self-worth; she experienced success that enabled her to feel in control of not only job seeking skills but also her goal to achieve independent living (Kavanagh & Fares, 1995). Creating a goal that was meaningful to Amy and could be achieved in a short time period appeared to enhance her self-worth, confidence, and abilities (Lindsey, 2000; MacKnee & Mervyn, 2002). At the time of discharge, Amy had begun to trust her abilities and believe in herself, and was scheduled to begin classes needed to complete her G.E.D. Amy and her therapist had set achievable goals and she was given the tools to take the steps needed to attain these goals. Amy's comments after just one month of occupational therapy intervention was, "The world has tried to push and shove me down but I am coming up and saying, watch out world here I come."

While Amy had the volitional intent and motivation needed to live independently, Carrie struggled with finding meaning in her life and could not identify personal interests, with the exception of being a good parent.

Baumann (1993) discusses how lack of self-determination was a common frustration among individuals living in the shelter setting because they felt that they could not independently determine the course of their lives. Carrie experienced this frustration because she perceived that the shelter staff was making her goals for her and determining how she would spend each day. These goals did not align with Carrie's personal goals. During the occupational therapy intervention, Carrie created goals with her therapist that met her own values, interests, and plans for her life and that of her son, instead of only meeting the goals that others had previously set for her. It is vital to have clients in a shelter population see the relevance of the goals in order for them to internalize them and truly make them their own to pursue (Sumsion, 2004). In addition, open communication at the client's level of understanding makes an important impact on developing goals. Carrie was able to make progress in forming goals relevant to her and attainable for her because of the open communication between client and therapist. It became apparent that incorporating Carrie's son into her goals was an important variable that was not initially considered.

Reciprocity greatly affects one's volition in the role of parent. The ability to effectively care for a child and have that child positively respond to that caring serves to reinforce the efficacy of the parental role. This feeling of reciprocity is vital to the mother-child relationship because it is affirming to both roles. Amy was concerned with her son and her ability to parent. Living in the shelter provided added stress to the relationship due to external rules and public parenting. By providing intervention to both Amy and her son, the therapist was able to prevent further decline in her son's development and their relationship (Hausman & Hammen, 1993). On the other hand, Carrie and her son demonstrated reciprocity in which both parent and child benefited. Even at a young age, Carrie's son was making eye contact and engaging positively with his mother, therefore he encouraged her role as parent. This was identified as an indication of Carrie's success as a mother utilizing a strength-based intervention strategy (Lindsey, 2000).

Habituation

The development of positive habits and routines also differed between Amy and Carrie. Habituation is "an internalized readiness to exhibit consistent patterns of behavior guided by our habits and roles and fitted to the characteristics of routine, temporal, physical, and social environments" (Kielhofner, 2002, p. 22). By discharge, Amy had begun to form positive habits in her life, including using a day planner and arriving on-time to appointments. It was reported by her case manager that she had made great gains in her ability to follow through with her commitments and responsibilities as well as arrive on-time to appointments. However, when there were an increased number of stressors in her life, such as being turned down for a permanent housing option, Amy's time management skills diminished. This indicated that skills had been developed but not converted to habits (Rogers, 2000). Although these time management skills diminished for brief periods of time, they did not cease because reinforcement of these skills and support to foster the formation of habits were provided during subsequent occupational therapy intervention sessions as well as by her case manager. The shelter staff also noted that Amy and her partner had received fewer reports for fighting and disobeying shelter rules during the period of time when occupational therapy intervention services were provided. Amy's ability to form new habits may have also been supported by the positive encouragement that she was receiving from her partner and son.

Carrie struggled to create meaningful habits for both her son and herself. It has been noted the importance of creating routines for families and their far reaching effects in the development of the child (Denham, 1995). One impoverished habit addressed was Carrie's inability to keep her son on a consistent schedule and sleeping in his crib during the night. A goal identified by Carrie was creating a sleep schedule and routine in which her son would sleep in his crib during the night. During intervention Carrie would discuss its importance and the safety benefits of this goal. Carrie reported making attempts to establish this routine, but her son only slept in his crib the entire night on two occasions. When probed as to the reason she did not meet this goal, Carrie stated that she would have her son sleep beside her when he first fell asleep and then she was too tired to lift him from the bed and place him in the crib positioned next to her bed. This reflects that Carrie had difficulties integrating her volitional intent with her ability to form meaningful habits and routines to meet her goals.

Performance Capacity

Performance capacity is defined as "the ability for doing things provided by the status of underlying objective physical and mental components and corresponding subjective experience" (Kielhofner, 2002, p. 24). Throughout intervention these underlying physical and mental components were seen as playing a vital role in the development of the intervention plan and ability to meet the stated goals of each mother. Amy was previously diagnosed with learning disabilities which made it necessary to simplify all discussions, make directions clear and concrete, and use simple vocabulary during intervention sessions. Although the results of the BDI indicated probable depression, depression did not appear to hinder Amy's ability to meet her goals. Amy was obese, but this physical component did not appear to affect her progress. Carrie's physical component of pain negatively affected her subjective experience in that it compromised her ability to engage in meaningful occupations. Carrie was overweight and she stated this caused her back pain. This back pain had far-reaching effects and, along with depression and decreased energy, greatly affected Carrie's ability to meet her goals. For example, Carrie had difficulties maintaining a consistent daily routine and attributed this to decreased energy.

CONCLUSIONS

In summary, the formation of achievable goals that are aligned with the client's own interests is necessary to achieve positive outcomes when working with homeless mothers living in a shelter (Brown & Bowen, 1998; Lindsey, 2000). The difference in outcomes between Carrie and Amy demonstrates how volition, habituation, and performance capacity play a role in the ability to achieve goals. Occupational therapists need to be aware of these personal attributes and include them in goals when working with this population. It is important to incorporate the strengths of each client into the goals and intervention sessions as well as consider the person's weaknesses in order to achieve success and make the client feel masterful in their endeavors (Kavanagh & Fares, 1995; Kearney, 1991). Both mothers were able to make self-generated goals but their differences in volition, habituation and performance capacity impacted their ability to meet these goals. Occupational therapists understand the value in asking the client about her/his progress and the need for repetition to create new habits to achieve goals. The homeless shelter is an appropriate place for occupational therapists to extend their skills to a community in order to provide intervention to an underserved population.

There are several limitations to this study. No formal assessment was administered to the women at the time of discharge. The women were not contacted after discharge to determine if they had continued to establish goals and work towards meeting those goals. The data collected was limited to these two women and cannot readily be transferred to larger segments of the homeless population.

More research needs to be conducted to demonstrate the value of goal setting with the homeless population. The rising incidence of homeless families, specifically single-headed families, makes this topic of increasing importance to the profession of occupational therapy.

REFERENCES

Banyard, V. L. & Graham-Bermann, S.A. (1995). Building an empowerment policy paradigm: Self-reported strengths of homeless mothers. *American Journal of Orthopsychiatry, 65,* 479-490.

Baron, K., Kielhofner, G., Iyenger, A., Goldhammer, V., & Wolenski, J. (2002). *The Occupational Self Assessment (OSA)* (Version 2.1). Chicago, IL: Model of Human Occupation Clearinghouse, University of Illinois at Chicago.

Bassuk, E.L., Browne, A., & Buckner, J.C. (1996). Single mothers and welfare. *Scientific American, 275*(4), 60-77.

Baumann, S.L. (1993). The meaning of being homeless. *Scholarly Inquiry for Nursing Practice: An International Journal, 7,* 59-70.

Beck, A.T., Steer, R.A., & Brown, G.K. (1996). *Manual for the Beck Depression Inventory-II.* San Antonio, TX: The Psychological Corporation.

Bromley, D. (1989). *The case-study method in psychology and related disciplines.* New York, NY: John Wiley & Sons.

Brown, C. & Bowen, R.E. (1998). Including the consumer and environment in occupational therapy treatment planning. *The Occupational Therapy Journal of Research, 18*(1), 44-61.

Choi, N.G. & Snyder, L.J. (1999). *Homeless families with children: A subjective experience of homelessness.* New York, NY: Springer Publ. Co.

Davis, J. & Kutter, C.J. (1998). Independent living skills and posttraumatic stress disorder in women who are homeless: Implications for future practice. *American Journal of Occupational Therapy, 52,* 39-44.

Denham, S.A. (1995). Family routines: A construct for considering family health. *Holistic Nursing Practce, 9*(4), 11-23.

DePoy, E. & Gitlin, L. (1998). *Introduction to research: Understanding and applying multiple strategies, 2nd Ed.* St. Louis, MO: Mosby.

Drake, M. (1992). Level I fieldwork in a daycare for homeless children. *Occupational Therapy in Health Care, 8,* 215-224.

Frankenburg, W.K., Dodds, J., Archer, P., Shapiro, H., & Bresnick, B. (1992). The Denver II: A major revision and restandardization of the Denver Developmental Screening Test. *Pediatrics, 89,* 91-96.

Hausman, B. & Hammen, C. (1993). Parenting in homeless families: The double crisis. *American Journal of Orthopsychiatry, 63,* 358-369.

Heubner, J. & Tryssenaar, J. (1996). Development of an occupational therapy practice perspective in a homeless shelter: A fieldwork experience. *Canadian Journal of Occupational Therapy, 63,* 24-32.

Kavanagh, J. & Fares, J. (1995). Using the model of human occupation with homeless mentally ill clients. *British Journal of Occupational Therapy, 58,* 419-422.

Kearney, P.C. (1991). Occupational therapy intervention with homeless women. *Occupational Therapy Practice, 2*(4), 75-81.

Kielhofner, G. (2002). Motives, patterns, and performance of occupation: Basic concepts. In G. Kielhofner (Ed.) *A Model of Human Occupation: Theory and application, 3rd ed.* (pp. 13-27). Maryland: Lippincott, Williams & Wilkins.

Kielhofner, G. & Forsyth, K. (2002). Therapeutic strategies for enabling change. In G. Kielhofner (Ed.) *A Model of Human Occupation: Theory and application, 3rd ed.* (pp. 309-324). Maryland: Lippincott, Williams & Wilkins.

Landry, J.E. (2001). Nobody told me it would be like this: The trials and triumphs of a research journey. In J.V. Cook (Ed.) *Qualitative research in occupational therapy* (pp. 98-112). Albany, NY: Delmar.

Lindsey, E.W. (2000). Social work with homeless mothers: A strength-based solution-focused model. *Journal of Family Social Work, 4*(1), 59-78.

MacKnee, C.M. & Mervyn, J. (2002). Critical incidence that facilitate homeless people's transition off the streets. *Journal of Social Distress and the Homeless, 11*(4), 293-306.

Menke, E.M. & Wagner, J.D. (1997). The experience of homeless female-headed families. *Issues in Mental Health Nursing, 18*, 315-330.

National Coalition for the Homeless (2004, May). *Facts about homelessness.* Retrieved September 11, 2005, from http://nationalhomeless.org/facts.html

Occupational Therapy Practice Framework: Domain and process. *American Journal of Occupational Therapy, 56*, 609-639.

Rogers, J. (2000). Habits: Do we practice what we preach? *Occupational Therapy Journal of Research, 20, Supplement 1,* 119s-137s.

Schultz-Krohn, W. (2004). Meaningful family routines in a homeless shelter. *American Journal of Occupational Therapy, 58*, 531-542.

Stake, R. (1994). Case studies. In N. Denzin & Y. Lincoln (Eds.) *Handbook of qualitative research* (pp. 236-247). Thousand Oaks, CA: Sage Publ.

Sumsion, T. (2004). Pursuing the client's goals really paid off. *British Journal of Occupational Therapy, 67*, 2-9.

Thrasher, S.P. & Mowbray, C.T. (1995). A strengths perspective: An ethnographic study of homeless women with children. *National Association of Social Workers, 20*, 93-101.

Townsend, E. & Wilcock, A.A. (2004). Occupational justice and client-centered practice: A dialogue in progress. *Canadian Journal of Occupational Therapy, 71*(2), 75-87.

Tryssenaar, J., Jones, E.J., & Lee, D. (1999). Occupational performance needs of a shelter population. *Canadian Journal of Occupational Therapy, 66*, 188-196.

Turner, S.M. (2004). *Homeless in America: How could it happen here?* Farmington Hills, MI: Thomsen.

Urban Institute, The (2000). *A new look at homelessness in America.* Retrieved September 8, 2005, from www.urban.org.

US Conference of Mayors (2003). *A status report on hunger and homelessness in America's cities: 2003.* Washington, DC: Author.

Yin, R. (2003). *Case study research: Design and methods, 3rd ed.* Thousand Oaks, CA: Sage Publ.

doi:10.1300/J003v20n03_10

Building Productive Roles: Occupational Therapy in a Homeless Shelter

Jaime Phillip Muñoz, PhD, OTR, FAOTA
Sara Dix, MOT, OTR/L
Diana Reichenbach, MOT, OTR/L

SUMMARY. Project Employ is a grant-funded program providing occupational therapy services to persons who are homeless. At Project Employ productive role involvement is the primary program outcome. Choices for productive role involvement are keyed by the person's interests and preferences, assessment is an ongoing process, prevocational training and rapid job placement are both available, and support and

Jaime Phillip Muñoz is Assistant Professor, Duquesne University, Department of Occupational Therapy. Sara Dix is Occupational Therapist, Project Employ, and Bethlehem Haven, Practice Scholar, Duquesne University, Department of Occupational Therapy. Diana Reichenbach, Program Coordinator, Project Employ Bethlehem Haven, Practice Scholar, Duquesne University, Department of Occupational Therapy.

Address correspondence to: Jaime Phillip Muñoz, Assistant Professor, Duquesne University, Department of Occupational Therapy, 219 Health Science Building, Pittsburgh, PA 15282 (E-mail: munoz@duq.edu).

The authors are indebted to the following individuals who are just a few of the many collaborators whose support has ensured the success of Project Employ: Marilyn Sullivan, Bethlehem Haven Executive Director, Connie Lewski, Employment Specialist, Project Employ, Nicole Ford, Bethlehem Haven Data Base Manager, and members of the Rainbow Research Team including Anne Marie Witchger Hansen, MS, OTR/L, Teressa Garcia, OTS, and Joy Lisak, OTS, all of Duquesne University.

[Haworth co-indexing entry note]: "Building Productive Roles: Occupational Therapy in a Homeless Shelter." Muñoz, Jaime Phillip, Sara Dix, and Diana Reichenbach. Co-published simultaneously in *Occupational Therapy in Health Care* (The Haworth Press, Inc.) Vol. 20, No. 3/4, 2006, pp. 167-187; and: *Homelessness in America: Perspectives, Characterizations, and Considerations for Occupational Therapy* (ed: Kathleen Swenson Miller, Georgiana L. Herzberg, and Sharon A. Ray) The Haworth Press, Inc., 2006, pp. 167-187. Single or multiple copies of this article are available for a fee from The Haworth Document Delivery Service [1-800-HAWORTH, 9:00 a.m. - 5:00 p.m. (EST). E-mail address: docdelivery@haworthpress.com].

Available online at http://othc.haworthpress.com
© 2006 by The Haworth Press, Inc. All rights reserved.
doi:10.1300/J003v20n03_11

work-place interventions, while not unlimited, can continue for up to two years. This article describes the process of assessing factors that act as supports or barriers to productive role functioning and shares intervention methods that support role competence and adaptation in this vulnerable population. doi:10.1300/J003v20n03_11 *[Article copies available for a fee from The Haworth Document Delivery Service: 1-800-HAWORTH. E-mail address: <docdelivery@haworthpress.com> Website: <http://www.HaworthPress.com>* *© 2006 by The Haworth Press, Inc. All rights reserved.]*

KEYWORDS. Supported employment, homelessness, COPM

INTRODUCTION

A focus on productivity has been part of the professional culture of occupational therapy since its inception. Indeed, over 80 years ago, Adolf Meyer proposed that a human's need for purposeful activity permeated the core of our being when he stated, "it is the use that we make of ourselves that gives the ultimate stamp to our every organ" (1922, p. 3). More recently, the Occupational Therapy Practice Framework (AOTA, 2002) explicitly identified work as an area of occupation in the professions' domain of practice. In this framework, work can be paid or unpaid and is inclusive of volunteer exploration and participation. The nature of work and its influence on occupation and personal identity is beginning to receive more focused attention from occupational therapy researchers (Primeau, 1996a, 1996b). Being employed not only puts bread on the table, but also helps people generate a sense of connectedness, of belonging and status, and of personal self-worth (Dickie, 2003; Kennedy-Jones, Cooper & Fossey, 2005). The purpose of this article is to add to the body of knowledge occupational therapists have about the nature of work and other productive roles with homeless populations, to describe the process of assessing factors that act as supports or barriers to productive role functioning, and to share intervention methods that support role competence and adaptation in this vulnerable population.

Employment Training Programs for Homeless

People who are homeless often present with a variety of problems that influence their capacity to secure and maintain employment. Some of these issues include deficiencies in basic living skills, a lack of transportation, mental illness, and addiction (U.S. Department of Labor, 1997). Other barriers to employment include a lack of education, a lack of personal identification documents, and limited competitive work skills (National Coalition for the Homeless, 1999). Nonetheless, not every person who is homeless is unemployed. The National Coalition for the Homeless (2001) estimates that more than one in four are employed usually in unskilled positions offering low wages, minimal job security, and no health benefits.

The U.S. Department of Labor (1997) created a best practices guide by culling together reports from over 63 organizations providing comprehensive services to persons and families who were homeless. This report suggested that the most effective programs were structured around one core agency that provided a variety of primary services including case management, counseling, vocational evaluation, job training services, job development and placement services, post-placement support services, housing, and life skills training. An essential component to successful programs was a strong network of linkages to other community services that could help a homeless person secure and retain employment. Many of these proposed best practice service components fall within the domain of occupational therapy.

Vocational Rehabilitation and Occupational Therapy

Work programming has been a component of occupational therapy since its inception as a profession (Jacobs, 1991). It is an approach grounded in moral treatment, exercised with soldiers returning from World War I, and energized with the passing of the vocational rehabilitation legislation (e.g., the Vocational Rehabilitation Act of 1920 and Vocational Rehabilitation Amendment of 1943) and the movement toward industrial rehabilitation in the 1960s (Auerbach & Jeong, 2005). Descriptions of occupational therapy work programming for persons with mental illnesses became more frequent in the 1980s. Initially, programs employing vocational rehabilitation strategies for use in inpatient psychiatric units were described in the literature (Palmer, 1982, 1985; Snyder, 1985). In the 1990s an increasing number of the vocational programs were community-based, such as the community work adjustment program described by Vanier (1991), programs emphasizing linkages with community supports programs (Lloyd & Basset, 1997), and vocational exploration groups for outpatients with psychiatric illnesses (Diamond, 1998). In general, these programs advocated thorough assessment of work skills, training to support the development of work skills, and definitions of vocational outcomes that included volunteerism, sheltered employment, transitional and supported employment, and competitive employment.

Best Practice Vocational Interventions

Some in the profession have recently argued that occupational therapy must examine best practice models for vocational rehabilitation (Auerbach & Jeong, 2005; Davis & Rinaldi, 2004; Moll, Huff & Detwiler, 2003). Moll and colleagues (2003) have argued that the Individual Placement and Supports model (Bond, 1998) is an evidenced-based vocational intervention that is compatible with the philosophical values and domain of practice of occupational therapy. The six principles of Individual Placement and Supports (IPS) model state that (1) competitive employment is the primary goal; (2) prevocational training is minimized in favor of rapid job placement; (3) vocational rehabilitation is integrated with other mental health services; (4) employment is keyed by the person's interests and preferences; (5) assessment is an ongoing process of establishing whether a fit exists between the person and the job environment, and (6) support and workplace interventions are time unlimited (Bond, 1998). The IPS model has good empirical support, but it may be less useful with people who are unable or unwilling to seek competitive employment (Auerbach, 2001).

This paper provides a description of an occupational therapy program for persons who are homeless that addresses both the needs of those seeking competitive employment and those who are unwilling or unable to do so. In this program productive role involvement replaces competitive employment as a primary goal for some participants and prevocational training and rapid job placement are both available. Like an ISP program, vocational rehabilitation in Project Employ is integrated with many other services that address the complex issues surrounding homelessness. Choices for productive role involvement are keyed by the person's interests and preferences, assessment is an ongoing process of establishing a person-environment fit, and support and workplace interventions, while not unlimited, can continue for up to two years.

PROJECT EMPLOY

Origins of the Program

Project Employ is a community-university partnership between a non-profit organization serving people who are homeless and an occupational therapy department at an Eastern private university. It is a grant-funded occupational therapy program aimed at providing homeless and formerly homeless individuals with individualized one-on-one and group services related to obtaining and maintaining meaningful and productive occupations. An occupational therapist has served as the director of the Project Employ program since 2001, but the seeds of the collaboration began when the Department of Occupational Therapy at Duquesne University created a Practice Scholar Program in 1999.

The occupational therapy department committed one faculty member's time for two years to collaborate with community agencies and create opportunities for students to connect curriculum content, service learning, and fieldwork education with "best practice" models in emerging community-based practice areas. The faculty member collaborated with the Executive Director of Bethlehem Haven to design a best practice occupational therapy program and to seek external funding to support this program. At this time, Project Employ was a vocationally-oriented program that lacked consistent structure and it became a focus of the community-university collaboration efforts. A proposal was submitted to the City of Pittsburgh and the Allegheny County Department of Human Services in response to a request for proposals that offered grant support to employment programs targeting homeless and incarcerated populations. In 2001, an initial three-year grant was awarded to the Department of Occupational Therapy at Duquesne University which included funding for a full-time occupational therapist to serve as the Project Employ Director. Since then, the Allegheny County Department of Human Services has continued to fund this program and additional grant funding has been secured from the U.S. Department of Health and Human Services as well as from local foundations. Over the past four years, Project Employ staff have developed and implemented new programming ideas to facilitate Project Employ's evolution from a non-structured weekly group session into a best practice model for occupational therapy programming with homeless populations.

The Setting

Bethlehem Haven is a non-profit organization located in downtown Pittsburgh that provides an array of vital health-care and social services under one roof. Health-care services provided at Bethlehem Haven include medical, podiatry, gynecological, and dental care. Individuals in need of mental health services can receive individual or group therapy. Legal advice and representation is available for individuals requiring assistance in civil cases such as child custody, bankruptcy, or divorce proceedings.

Bethlehem Haven operates an emergency overnight shelter and three other residential programs for homeless women. The 32-bed overnight shelter provides housing, meals, and intensive case management services. Two of the three residential programs are designed to serve women dealing with substance abuse issues. The STAR (Striving Toward Authentic Recovery) Program accommodates 10 women in early stages of recovery. Women in the STAR program are provided with housing for up to four months. They share double-occupancy rooms, prepare and take meals in a common kitchen area, and participate in intensive case management services. Women who are further along in their recovery process can be admitted to the Step-Up Program, a 10-bed transitional housing program. Women in the Step-Up Program live in private rooms for up to two years paying 30% of their income as a monthly program fee. With the support of program staff, women are encouraged to manage their time, budget their income, and actively participate in their own recovery. This program focuses on preparing women for reentry into independent community living.

The newest residential program is the SOAR (Safe Oasis and Residence) Program. SOAR is a 16-bed safe haven. A safe haven is a type of supportive housing designed to serve chronically homeless persons with severe and persistent mental illnesses who have been unwilling or unable to participate in support services (HUD, 2001). The SOAR Program at Bethlehem Haven provides 16 women with private rooms and a consistent home-like environment. The focus of the SOAR program is to provide stable housing and opportunities for residents to engage in typical daily activities. Supportive services emphasize harm reduction and motivational engagement. However, in keeping with safe haven principles, these supportive programs are made available and encouraged but a resident's participation is not mandatory.

The Population

To qualify for enrollment in a Project Employ program a person must be at least 18 years old, be currently or formerly homeless, and must express a willingness to work or to maintain a productive occupational role. If an enrollee is receiving substance abuse and/or mental health treatment, Project Employ requires ongoing verification that the enrollee is continuing treatment. In the last fiscal year, 97 people enrolled in Project Employ programs. Approximately four out of five applicants were female (81%)

and most were black (65%). The mean age of enrollees was 40.5 years with a range from 21 to 61. Participants came to Project Employ with varied educational and vocational histories. Most applicants (69%) had high-school diplomas and a few (16.3%) had some college education. Most enrollees (94%) were unemployed and the average period of unemployment prior to enrollment was nearly two years. Those with employment histories reported holding jobs which required little or no formal training, paid low wages and offered no health benefits. Nearly two thirds (64%) held jobs paying $7.00 an hour or less and nearly all (95%) earned salaries that were below a living wage for the city of Pittsburgh which has been calculated at $10.39 plus benefits (Thomas Merton Center, 2005). Just over half of the enrollees (57%) reported that their only source of regular income was some form of public assistance (cash assistance, medical assistance, food stamps, SSI/SSDI).

The majority of the enrollees in Project Employ have histories of mental illness, addiction and criminality. Almost all of the applicants (92%) had participated in drug and alcohol recovery programs in the past and four out of five (81%) of these were participating in drug treatment programs at the time of their enrollment. Two thirds of the respondents (66%) had received mental health services in the past and most of these (59%) continued to receive these services at the time of their enrollment. The most common psychiatric diagnosis reported by enrollees was depression, followed by bipolar and anxiety disorders. Most applicants (80.4%) reported a criminal history.

Initial Assessment and Placement

Participation in Project Employ is mandatory for women in Bethlehem Haven's STAR and Step-Up programs, and in the last fiscal year the majority of applicants (53%) came directly from one of these programs. One third (33%) of all applicants were referred by case managers from local shelters or transitional housing programs and the remaining enrollees (14%) were directed to Project Employ by their family, friends, or former graduates of the program.

Individuals who decide to pursue enrollment independently complete and submit an enrollment application. Enrollment begins with an occupational therapist using the person's completed application to initiate a screening interview. In addition to determining eligibility and answering an applicant's question about the programs, the therapist elicits and verifies information about the applicant's housing, income, educational and vocational history, substance use, medical and mental health history, criminal background, and family and social contexts. After this screening, the therapist recommends enrollment into Project Employ's Professional Development or Life Skills Program, or provides the applicant with referrals to other vocational and/or educational programs in the community.

Individuals in the STAR or Step-Up programs are automatically placed in the Life Skills program and make up the bulk of the enrollees to this program. Some of these individuals begin in Life Skills and transfer to Professional Development provided they meet the eligibility requirements and a new rotation of classes is beginning. To be eligible for the Professional Development program an applicant must have at least 60 days of clean time, must be engaged in mental health and/or addiction treatment (if applicable), and must express a clear desire to find productive employment. Applicants who want to work but cannot commit to addressing their mental health or addiction issues may enroll in Life Skills or may be referred to other programs in the community. Applicants who want to work but are concerned that working will jeopardize their social security benefits are referred to other programs and the local social security office with information about their Ticket to Work program (Social Security Online, 2005).

The occupational therapist and participant utilize initial sessions to complete the *Canadian Occupational Performance Measure* (COPM) and to develop individualized goal plans (Law et al., 2005). The COPM is typically completed within two weeks of enrollment into a program. The COPM supports a person-centered assessment process that encourages the participant to identify issues in occupational performance areas of self-care, productivity, leisure, and social participation (see Muñoz et al., this volume). Reevaluations using the COPM generally occur at three-month intervals to follow-up and monitor the person's progress. The therapist and participant use the COPM results to collaboratively develop an action plan to address the participant's self-identified goals. Goal writing is taught and regularly reinforced in classes and implemented during 1-on-1 sessions by utilizing the SMART acronym (specific, measurable, actionable, realistic, timely) to assist participants in developing and evaluating their goals.

Design Characteristics of the Programs

Although the Professional Development and Life Skills programs at Project Employ each have a distinct and separate focus (see Figure 1), they share some similar design characteristics. These include a heavy em-

FIGURE 1. Flow Chart of Occupational Therapy Services

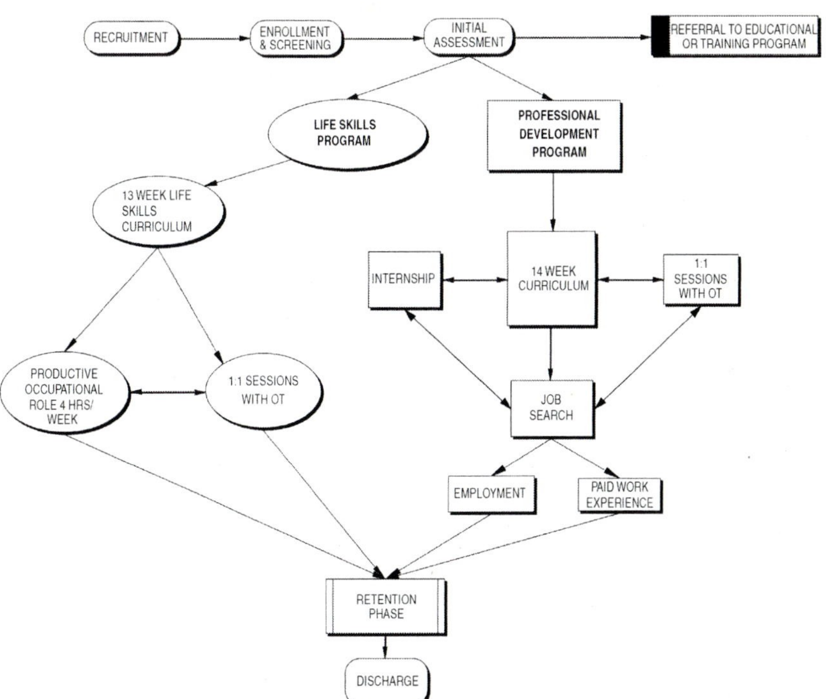

phasis on personally responsible behavior, a clear focus on the development of routines that support productive role performance, a defined set of curriculum topics, the use of the COPM to set and monitor goal attainment, and a reliance on interactive intervention strategies. Enrollees in both these programs are expected to attend all 1-on-1 sessions and every scheduled class, on time. During initial individual sessions with their occupational therapist, participants are provided assistance in obtaining personal documents including a birth certificate, photo identification, and a Social Security card since about half (56%) of the applicants are missing one or all of these forms of identification. Such documentation is frequently required in applications for employment, housing or training programs. Weekly individual meetings are an integral component of both programs. It is here that the therapist works to establish a trusting therapeutic relationship with the enrollee and creates an environment that supports honest dialogue and feedback, and where each can share feelings and concerns openly.

Over the four-plus years that Project Employ has included occupational therapy services, practitioners have learned that one key to shaping productive behavior is to have and enforce clear behavioral expectations for personal responsibility. Guidelines for attendance and punctuality are strictly enforced to facilitate good time management skills and instill personal habits of self-responsibility. No one is permitted into a class once it has begun unless prior arrangements for being late have been made. Participants who routinely demonstrate effective habits of personal responsibility are rewarded with a bus pass or other incentives each month. Other incentives, such as intermittently awarding small prizes to acknowledge class participation, random drawings for health and self-care products, tickets to amusement and theater events, and distributing vouchers to shop for professional clothing, are also effective reinforcers.

Practitioners have also learned that in order to increase motivation and combat the volitional deficits often seen in this population, participants need to be fully engaged in group learning processes. Group sessions in both programs are designed to be highly interactive. Dress for success sessions, mock interviewing, employer panel discussions and group field trips are examples of sessions that emphasize active participation. Group processes that have been found to be effective with this population include the use of icebreakers that emphasize socialization, self-esteem building, sensory stimulation and physical movement. Strategies for engaging the participants include using popular music, role playing, small group work, games, and competition with prizes when appropriate.

The Life Skills Program

Many of the enrollees in the Life Skills (LS) program are in early stages of their recovery process. For the vast majority of these participants, working on recovery from addiction and stabilizing their mental health are primary goals and take precedence over employment. The primary outcome for participants in the LS program is to develop a skill set and an occupational performance pattern that support productive role involvement. Minimum program requirements for enrollees include attending one class each week and meeting individually once a week with their occupational therapist. Participants complete a 13-week sequence of classes. This series of classes repeats four times a year and an enrollee may enter the class rotation at any point in the sequence. Examples of topics covered in the LS program include time and stress management, conflict resolution, health and wellness, and goal setting. The full schedule of topics is presented in Table 1.

When participants have completed approximately two thirds of their LS classes they are expected to be spending four hours each week participating in a self-selected productive activity. Many choose to incorporate a volunteer position into their routine and enrollees have taken positions in hair salons, animal shelters, soup kitchens, or church meal programs. Others experiment with educational roles and take classes in computers, courses in preparation for acquiring their GED, or other certificate training programs. Once a participant has completed the full LS sequence and has incorporated a productive role activity they move into the retention phase of the program.

During the retention phase participants are expected to maintain four hours of productive role activity. The participant continues to meet weekly in 1:1 sessions with the occupational therapist to support continued participation in activities that support productive role functioning. In these individual sessions the COPM provides the structure for identifying problems, monitoring progress and establishing new goals. Participants continue in the retention phase as long as they are living in one of Bethlehem Haven's residential programs or up to six months after they have moved on to other housing.

TABLE 1. Life Skills Program Curriculum

Week	Class
1	I Know I Can!
2	Explore Your Interests
3	Interest Presentations
4	SMART Goals
5	Effective Communication
6	Time Management
7	Stress Management
8	Anger Management & Conflict Resolution
9	Making Good Decisions
10	Change–Deal With It!
11	Money Talks
12	Transitioning Into Independence
13	Health & Wellness

In the past fiscal year, 62% of the enrollees in the LS program completed the curriculum. The majority of those unable to complete the program were unsuccessful secondary to a relapse of their addiction or mental illness. Others were unable to comply with Bethlehem Haven behavioral guidelines for maintaining residency. Of those who did complete the program, 65% engaged in educational or volunteer activities and 42% found employment to meet their expectations for productive role activity. Many graduates of the Life Skills program (42%) successfully enrolled in the Professional Development program.

Caroline: Finding Meaning Through Productive Activity

Many of the women in Bethlehem Haven's residential programs are initially resistant to becoming involved in a vocational activity. Some of the causes for this resistance can be a lack of motivation, a lack of insight into their vocational interests, not wanting to "take the focus off of their recovery," a fear of taking on new challenges, or feeling incapable or inadequate. The following is a story of one woman's journey to leading a meaningful and productive life. Her story begins with an expectation to engage in productive activity.

Caroline enrolled in the LS program when she entered the STAR program at Bethlehem Haven. Using the COPM, Caroline identified primary goals of staying clean and sober, maintaining her mental health, obtaining permanent housing, and eventually getting a job. Caroline had no specialized training or education beyond high school, but expressed an interest in learning more about computers. She enrolled in a six-week computer basics class offered at Project Employ that allowed her to explore this interest and meet her program requirement of involvement in professional role activity for four hours a week.

As the completion of her computer course neared, Caroline expressed an interest in becoming involved in an activity where she could help others in the community. Caroline and her therapist identified several potential volunteer sites and Caroline contacted each for information. This process led her to pursue a 14-week volunteer training course for a crisis hotline at a local women's shelter. During the same time, Caroline responded to an advertised request for volunteers to assist with the operation of a cold weather shelter in Pittsburgh. Within a short time, Caroline was not only volunteering at the shelter, but was also coordinating the meals program on a weekly basis. By the time the cold weather shelter had closed for the season, Caroline had completed her crisis hotline training and was ready to start volunteering at the women's shelter.

These activities helped Caroline recognize that she found meaning in her own life by helping others. Caroline decided to investigate requirements for pursuing a drug and alcohol counseling certificate. With her therapist's support she completed the college enrollment process and began full-time classes at the local community college in the fall of 2005. As of this writing, Caroline is attending full-time college classes and continues to volunteer regularly at the women's crisis center and at Bethlehem Haven's SOAR program. She is planning to move into her own apartment soon. Her goals now include completing her college certificate program, continuing to volunteer, and obtaining full-time employment working in a social service setting.

The Professional Development Program

Unlike the open enrollment of the Life Skills program, participants are admitted into the Professional Development (PD) program at the beginning of each new rotation of classes which occurs approximately every four months. This cohort model of enrollment is designed to facilitate group cohesiveness. Generally 15-20 enrollees are admitted into each new cohort and this group is divided into a morning and an evening class. The primary focus of the PD program is to assist individuals who are able and committed to becoming employed to secure and retain meaningful employment. Participants in this program are required to attend classes three days per week for 14 weeks. They devote time to completing employment oriented projects and homework outside of class including developing resumes and job application cover letters, preparing for class presentations, and completing job searching assignments. Topics covered in the PD curriculum are presented in Table 2. The level of material presented in classes is more complex, the frequency of class sessions is more intense, and the expectations for professional and self-directed behavior are much higher in this program than in the Life Skills program.

Job Searching

An enrollee in the PD program can initiate a job search at any point in the program. While participants share a common goal of competitive employment, they come to the program with varied levels of education and vocational histories, work adjustment skills, and self-confidence. The degree to which participants feel compelled by their current life circumstances to find employment and earn an income immediately also varies considerably. Although rare, some participants are already employed

TABLE 2. Professional Development Program Curriculum

Week	Class	Class	Class
1	I Know I Can!	Explore Your Interests	Identify Your Skills
2	Winning Resumes	SMART Goals	Career Presentations
3	Resume Workshop	Resume Workshop	Finding the Job That Fits
4	Dress For Success *Field Trip*	Finding Employment With a Criminal Record	Presentations
5	Testing the Waters–Internships	Sell Yourself at an Interview–Part 1	Selling Yourself at an Interview–Part 2
6	Sell Yourself at an Interview–Part 3	Time Management	Cover Letters & Thank You Notes
7	Cover Letter Writing Workshop	Manage Your Stress	**NO CLASS!**
8	The Application Process (in person)	Anger & Conflict Management	The Application Process (online)
9	Professionally Speaking	Decision Making	Money Talks–Part 1
10	Job Fair Etiquette & Networking	Change–Deal With It!	Money Talks–Part 2
11	FIELD TRIP (to be announced)	Transitioning Into Independence	FIELD TRIP (to be announced)
12	Employer Panel Discussions	Relapse Prevention	Employer Panel Discussions
13	Job Search (if job not yet obtained)	Dining With Class	Job Search (if job not yet obtained)
14	Internship Wrap-up & Presentations	Health & Wellness	Class Certificates & Awards

when they enter the program and a primary goal they may have is to find a better paying job that offers health benefits. The occupational therapists work closely with the employment specialist to assist the participants involved in job searching. In classes, participants identify their areas of vocational interest through various group and self-reflection activities, and through internship and volunteer opportunities. In individual meetings the occupational therapist helps the participant evaluate their past work, educational or training experiences, and their strengths for and barriers to employment. Career assessments such as *The Job Search Attitude Inventory* and the *Barriers to Employment Success Inventory* may be utilized while *The Career Exploration Inventory* is administered with every participant.

Participants are taught job searching strategies and encouraged to use a variety of methods in their job search including newspaper and internet searching, using local CareerLink programs, attending job fairs and networking with others. Project Employ also maintains a Job Board where employment opportunities are posted. Through continuous networking with personnel managers at local businesses, the employment specialist and Project Employ staff have created the types of relationships where employers will independently notify Project Employ staff of job openings in their businesses. Human resource managers and business owners also support the job searching process by participating directly in the PD classes. They may assist in resume and cover letter writing workshops, play the role of the personnel manager in mock interviewing sessions or participate in question and answer sessions or panel discussions. This collaboration is an intentional design of the program. It offers the participants a direct networking opportunity while also providing potential employers the opportunity to familiarize themselves with the rigors and professionalism of the program and the participants' abilities to meet their high expectations. It also creates an opportunity for cross-cultural encounters which help the employers expand their understanding of the complexity of issues surrounding homelessness and to confront stereotypes they may have about individuals who are homeless.

Internship Placements

In their 7th week of the curriculum, every participant who has not secured employment begins an unpaid eight-week internship. Participants are provided with a list of 25-30 different internship positions to choose from. They select three positions to interview for and independently schedule and complete the interviews. They process these experiences with the occupational therapist and employment specialist and choose the internship that offers the best fit for them. The participant works four hours a week in an internship placement designed as an opportunity for enrollees to demonstrate work and professional behaviors in an authentic work environment. For example, participants have completed internships in local banks, hospitals, day programs for adults with disabilities, libraries, food banks, retail settings, and clerical and cleaning positions. These internships provide an opportunity for enrollees to build self-confidence and gain a deeper understanding of themselves as workers. Almost all of the interns are able to secure a solid, recent reference from their internship supervisors to use in subsequent job interviews. Supervisors complete written evaluations during the 2nd, 4th and 8th week of the internship. Several interns have secured jobs by being encouraged to apply for positions in other departments within the same organization. Those who have already found work by the 7th week are not required to complete an internship, although some voluntarily choose to do so.

Paid Work Experiences

Project Employ has contracted with several local employers to provide Paid Work Experiences (PWEs) for participants who are experiencing exceptional difficulty in securing stable employment. PWEs are part time (20-24 hrs/week) positions that have been created in dietary, environmental, clerical, retail, and warehouse settings. The occupational therapists and employment specialist refer participants for these positions after carefully considering workplace demands and an individual's work adjustment skills and attitudes. Once referred, the participant completes the company's normal interviewing and orientation process. If the person is hired, Project Employ pays the participant's salary (up to 24 hours/week). The PWE can last for up to six months. The ultimate goal of the PWE placement is for participants to be considered for hire as permanent staff by the respective employers. Project Employ staff try to facilitate this outcome by working closely with the participants and their supervisors to address job-related or personal issues that arise. Job performance evaluations are completed by the supervisors and reviewed with the participant at one, three, and six month intervals. Project Employ staff also review the evaluations with the participant to ensure their full comprehension of the feedback. Staff also complete on-site visits, attend meetings with participants and their supervisors if requested, and continue 1-on-1 meetings at Project Employ throughout the PWE. The PWE approach has been very successful. To date, nine of 12 participants who have completed a PWE (75%) were hired by their respective PWE employers. Among the three who were not hired, one individual left the PWE due to a chronic illness, another left after experiencing a relapse in addiction and the third was unsuccessful secondary to an exacerbation of mental illness.

Job Retention

In the PD Program the length of the retention period varies depending on the participant's success in securing competitive employment. If a participant has not secured employment after completing the PD curriculum, the occupational therapists and employment specialist work intensively with the person to update goals particularly around the job searching process. The participant and Project Employ staff typically generate a behavioral schedule for specific job search activities. Measurable goals may include the number or hours and/or days a week that the participant will spend on-site in a job search process. Specifying the expectations for the number of applications or resumes to be submitted each week or the number of follow-up phone calls to companies where applications were submitted that will be made are not unusual. The participant is also required to complete and update a job search tracking tool that was developed by Project Employ staff to organize and document the participant's job search efforts.

Participants who become employed during or after completing the PD curriculum also receive support services to facilitate the person's success in job retention and to encourage advancement. These services can be provided for up to 12 months after the person is employed. Continued follow-up and the maintenance of an ongoing trusting relationship with the participant during job retention are essential. Oftentimes a participant's initial response to job stress may be to resort to old behaviors (anger, avoidance, substance use) leading to job loss. During this time participants continue to meet with the occupational therapist once a month to discuss their worker role and the integration of this new role into their lives. In these retention meetings the therapist and participant may problem-solve issues that could interfere with job retention (e.g., child care, transportation, housing, mental health or substance abuse treatment, etc.). Job-related or performance issues such as not getting along with supervisors or coworkers or a reduction in work hours are also topics that may arise.

After a period of work adjustment, participants are encouraged to think about ways they can further develop their worker role. Options for advancement may include seeking increased wages or hours, working towards a promotion to a new position or department, or accepting additional responsibilities. If advancement is identified as a personal goal, the therapist and enrollee identify strategies to realize this goal. Strategies may include making a request for continuing education or training, initiating a discussion with the supervisor about opportunities for advancement, monitoring internal job postings, applying for different positions, or volunteering to stay late at work when needed. The results of their efforts are discussed during their follow-up sessions to determine or to celebrate the effectiveness of these approaches or to consider adaptations or additional measures that can be taken.

In the past fiscal year, the majority of the enrollees (35/50; 70%) who entered the Professional Development program successfully completed the curriculum. The reasons for not completing the curriculum are varied, but include relapses of addiction or mental illness, obtaining employment and choosing not to continue the PD classes, relocation, or being unable or unwilling to meet program requirements. Of those who completed the full PD curriculum the majority (28/35; 80%) found employment within six weeks of completion. Five other individuals who began, but did not complete, the curriculum found employment. Many of the PD graduates (40%) not only found employment, but also participated in some type of educational or vocational training program such as computer training, enrolling in certificate programs for drug and alcohol counseling, horticultural training, commercial drivers license training, culinary, floral arranging, or GED classes. Two graduates are pursuing associate degrees in criminal justice and library sciences respectively.

Joe: Getting a Life Back on Track

The following account is one of engineering hope in a man who had been hopeless. Perseverance, dedication, and hard work nurtured with guidance and ongoing support of the Project Employ staff are key themes that play out in this and many of the participants' stories. Joe came to the PD program with a lengthy history of drug addiction and homelessness, and a spotty work history. Joe could secure but could not retain employment and his work adjustment problems were typically centered on his addiction. Despite this past history, Joe had many strengths. He had graduated from high school, had taken some college courses, and had held a variety of jobs in the past including positions in health care, hospitality and in environmental services. Joe did not have a criminal record, had several months of clean time and expressed a strong motivation to get his life "back on track." His personal goals were to find a stable full-time job, get off of welfare, save some money, and get his own apartment.

Joe participated readily and had perfect attendance in the Professional Development classes. His performance evaluations from his internship as an aide in the recovery room at a local hospital were all in the very-good to excellent range. As Joe neared the completion of the PD curriculum, he worked diligently with the occupational therapist and the employment specialist to plan out his job search strategy. Within a few weeks he had secured a job in the housekeeping department of a local hospital working full-time for $7.25 an hour with medical benefits. Joe was happy with this new job, but soon realized that he wanted more, and more importantly, he believed he was capable of more. During his job retention monthly meetings, Joe reexamined his goals for self-sufficiency and he established a new goal plan focusing on job retention and wage advancement. Joe's strategies included maintaining his perfect work attendance record, covering extra shifts when asked, and obtaining information from his boss regarding the criteria for getting a pay raise. About the same time, Project Employ staff were asked for help finding a reliable individual to work in the housekeeping department of another hospital. While the position was only casual, it had the potential of going part-time or full-time and it paid between $10.25 and $15.00 per hour based on the shift differential.

Joe's schedule at his current job was steady and regular and he concluded that if he could work evening and weekend shifts for the second hospital he could earn more and get his foot in the door at a better paying job. Project Employ staff referred Joe for this position. The company was so impressed with Joe that they offered him the position the next day and Joe started working one to two shifts a week at the second hospital. Before long, Joe's willingness to work any shift, his job performance, and his attitude resulted in his being called to work even more shifts. He gave his first employer two weeks resignation notice and before long he was hired to a full-time position with good pay, full medical benefits, paid time off and overtime. During this time Joe continued to meet the requirements of the program, meeting at least monthly with the OT, attending 12-step meetings, and updating his goal plan as needed. At the time of this writing Joe had saved a significant amount of his earnings and was looking for his own apartment.

CONCLUSION

The purpose of this article is to describe the development, structure and outcomes of Project Employ, an occupational therapy program that engages homeless persons in the process of developing and maintaining worker and other productive occupational roles. Best practice interventions for populations who are homeless and mentally ill include promoting engagement; providing structured activities; and facilitating trusting relationships, expectations for self-responsibility, limit setting for destructive behaviors, and positive reinforcement, all of which are encompassed by occupational therapy philosophies. This paper presented a description of the methods used to facilitate holistic, occupation-based interventions in this setting and the clinical reasoning behind creating a best practice model in a community-based residential setting for persons who are homeless. The evolution of the program and mechanisms of funding were shared to encourage replication of similar programs. Occupational therapists are well-equipped for providing services to this marginalized population through person-centered interventions. A role for occupational therapy can be developed by creating population-based programs that focus on removing the barriers to self-sufficiency through life skills training, developing vocational roles, securing housing, and facilitating involvement in substance abuse and mental health treatment.

REFERENCES

American Occupational Therapy Association (2002). Occupational therapy practice framework: Domain and process. *American Journal of Occupational Therapy, 56*, 609-639.

Auerbach, E.S. (2001). The Individual Placement and Support Model vs. the Menu Approach to supported employment: Where does occupational therapy fit in? *Occupational Therapy in Mental Health, 17*, 2, 1-19.

Auerbach, E.S. & Jeong, G. (2005). Vocational programming. In E. Cara & A. MacRae (Eds.), *Psychosocial occupational therapy: A clinical practice*. 2nd edition. Clifton, NY: Thompson Delmar Learning.

Bond, G.R. (1998). Principles of the individual placement and support model: Empirical support. *Psychiatric Rehabilitation Journal, 22*, 11-23.

Davis, M. & Rinaldi, M. (2004). Using an evidence-based approach to enable people with mental health problems to gain and retain employment, education and voluntary work. *British Journal of Occupational Therapy, 67*, 7, 319-322.

Diamond, H. (1998). Vocational decision making in a psychiatric outpatient program. *Occupational Therapy in Mental Health, 14*, 3, 67-80.

Dickie, V.A. (2003). Establishing worker identity: A study of people in craft work. *American Journal of Occupational Therapy, 57*, 250-261.

Jacobs, K. (1991). *Occupational therapy: Work-related programs and assessments.* 2nd edition. Boston: Little, Brown and Company.

Kennedy-Jones, M., Cooper, J., & Fossey, E. (2005). Developing a worker role: Stories of four people with mental illness. *Australian Occupational Therapy Journal, 52*, 2, 116-126.

Law, M., Baptiste, S., Carswell, A., McColl, M.A., Polatajko, H., & Pollock, N. (2005). *Canadian occupational performance measure*, 4th edition. Ottawa: Canadian Association of Occupational Therapists, Inc.

Lloyd, C. & Basset, J. (1997). Life is for living: A prevocational programme for young people with psychosis. *Australian Occupational Therapy Journal, 44*, 2, 82-87.

Meyer, A. (1922). The philosophy of occupational therapy. *Archives of Occupational Therapy, 1*, 1-10.

Moll, S., Huff, J., & Detwiler, L. (2003). Supported employment: Evidence for a best practice model in psychosocial rehabilitation. *Canadian Journal of Occupational Therapy, 70*, 5, 298-310.

Muñoz, J., Garcia, T., Lisak, J. & Reichenbach, D. (2006). Assessing the Occupational Performance Priorities of People Who Are Homeless. *Occupational Therapy in Health Care,* this volume.

National Coalition for the Homeless (1999). *Homeless Fact Sheet #4: Employment and homelessness*. Retrieved June 30, 2004, from http://www.nationalhomeless.org/jobs.html

National Coalition for the Homeless. (2001). *Welfare to what? Available from the National Coalition for the Homeless, 1012 Fourteenth Street, NW, Suite 600, Washington, DC; 202/737-6444, www.nationalhomeless.org.*

Palmer, F. (1982). Transitional employment project. *Occupational Therapy in Mental Health, 2 , 2, 23-36.*

Palmer, F. (1985). Vocational treatment model. *Occupational Therapy in Mental Health, 5*, 1, 41-58.

Primeau, L. (1996a). Work and leisure: Transcending the dichotomy. *American Journal of Occupational Therapy, 50*, 569-577.

Primeau, L. (1996b). Work versus non-work: The case of household work. In R. Zemke & F. Clark (Eds.), *Occupational science: The evolving discipline* (pp. 57-70). Philadelphia: F. A. Davis.

Snyder, S. (1985). Comprehensive inpatient treatment for the young adult patient. *Occupational Therapy in Mental Health, 5*, 2, 47-58.

Social Security Online (2005). *Fact Sheet: Ticket to Work and Work Incentives Improvement Act of 1999*. Retrieved October 10, 2005, from: http://www.ssa.gov/work/ResourcesToolkit/legisregfact.html

Thomas Merton Center (2005). *What is a living wage in Allegheny County?* Accessed September 12, 2005, from http://www.thomasmertoncenter.org/laborpledge/moreinfo.htm

U.S. Department of Housing and Urban Development (2001). *Overview of the Supportive Housing Program: Program components*. Retrieved October 10, 2005 from http://www.hud.gov/offices/cpd/homeless/library/shp/understandingshp/components.cfm

U.S. Department of Labor (1997). *Employment and training for America's homeless: Best practices guide.*. Retrieved January 27, 2004 from http://www.doleta.gov/documents/homelessman/homeless.asp

Vanier, C. (1991). The community work project: An occupational therapy programme. *Canadian Journal of Occupational Therapy, 58*, 3, 123-128.

doi:10.1300/J003v20n03_11

Life Skill Interventions with Homeless Youth, Domestic Violence Victims and Adults with Mental Illness

Christine A. Helfrich, PhD, OTR/L
Ann M. Aviles, MS, OTR/L
Chaula Badiani, MS, OTR/L
Deborah Walens, MHPE, OTR/L
Peggy Sabol, MA, OTR/L

SUMMARY. This paper presents three exploratory studies of life skills interventions (employment, money management or food/nutrition) with 73 homeless individuals from four shelters and supportive housing pro-

---

Christine A. Helfrich is Assistant Professor, Department of Occupational Therapy, University of Illinois at Chicago M/C 811, 1919 West Taylor Street, Chicago, IL 60612-7250. Ann M. Aviles is Research Specialist in Health Sciences, Department of Psychiatry, University of Illinois at Chicago, 1747 W. Roosevelt Road, MC 747, RM 155, Chicago, IL 60612. Chaula Badiani is Staff Occupational Therapist, Innovative Pediatrics, L.L.C. in Chicago, 5315 N. Clark St #260, Chicago, IL 60640. This work was completed as a Research Assistant, Department of Occupational Therapy, University of Illinois at Chicago. Deborah Walens is Clinical Associate Professor, Department of Occupational Therapy, University of Illinois at Chicago. Peggy Sabol is Manager, Psychiatry, Stone Institute of Psychiatry, Northwestern Memorial Hospital, 446 E. Ontario, 7th floor, Room 246, Chicago, IL 60611.

This study was supported by grants from the Great Cities Faculty Seed Fund and the Campus Research Board at the University of Illinois at Chicago.

[Haworth co-indexing entry note]: "Life Skill Interventions with Homeless Youth, Domestic Violence Victims and Adults with Mental Illness." Helfrich, Christine A. et al. Co-published simultaneously in *Occupational Therapy in Health Care* (The Haworth Press, Inc.) Vol. 20, No. 3/4, 2006, pp. 189-207; and: *Homelessness in America: Perspectives, Characterizations, and Considerations for Occupational Therapy* (ed: Kathleen Swenson Miller, Georgiana L. Herzberg, and Sharon A. Ray) The Haworth Press, Inc., 2006, pp. 189-207. Single or multiple copies of this article are available for a fee from The Haworth Document Delivery Service [1-800-HAWORTH, 9:00 a.m. - 5:00 p.m. (EST). E-mail address: docdelivery@haworthpress.com].

Available online at http://othc.haworthpress.com
© 2006 by The Haworth Press, Inc. All rights reserved.
doi:10.1300/J003v20n03_12

grams located in the urban Midwest for youth, victims of domestic violence and adults with mental illness. The Ansell Casey Life Skills Assessment was administered prior to the eight group and individual sessions. Quizzes and posttests indicated clinical change in all groups, with statistical significance in the domestic violence group. The intervention implementation, challenges encountered, and strategies developed for implementing shelter-based interventions are discussed. Recommendations for successfully providing collaborative university-shelter clinical interventions are provided. doi:10.1300/J003v20n03_12 *[Article copies available for a fee from The Haworth Document Delivery Service: 1-800-HAWORTH. E-mail address: <docdelivery@haworthpress.com> Website: <http://www.HaworthPress.com> © 2006 by The Haworth Press, Inc. All rights reserved.]*

KEYWORDS. Homelessness, mental illness, domestic violence, youth, life skills

INTRODUCTION AND LITERATURE REVIEW

Homeless individuals present diverse life skill needs related to living independently. In addition to poverty, homeless individuals identify occupational performance problems related to finances, housing, personal care, difficulties satisfying basic needs, and health concerns (Tryssenaar, Jones, & Lee, 1999). The experience of homelessness is often complicated by a variety of unique physical (Substance Abuse and Mental Health Services Administration, 2003) and mental disorders (First, Rife, & Kraus, 1990; Folsom & Jeste, 2002). Homelessness itself is a risk factor for emotional disorders (Goodman, Saxe, & Harvey, 1991). In combination, these physical and mental sequelae place the individual at risk for functional impairments that necessitate institutional care. The occupational therapy literature has demonstrated the need for, and effectiveness of, life skills interventions with homeless individuals in shelters (Davis, Hagen, & Early, 1994; Gutmann, 1975; C. A. Helfrich, 2001; Kannenberg, 1997; Shordike, 2001; Tryssenaar, Jones, & Lee, 1999). The limited research on the effectiveness of life skills programs for homeless individuals indicates much more is needed. This paper describes exploratory interventions with three groups: (1) homeless youth without families (employment skills), (2) women fleeing abusive homes (managing finances), and (3) persons with mental illnesses (securing and managing food).

Youth

Youth homelessness in the United States has become an epidemic with estimates reaching as high as two million (Ensign, 1998). In 2004, children under 18 years accounted for 39% of the urban homeless population (National Coalition for the Homeless). Some of these youths have children of their own, placing their children and themselves at risk. These youths may acquire survival skills while living on the street but they do not develop the life skills needed to become independent, self-supporting adults who are integrated into the larger society.

Adolescents who are homeless often leave abusive and neglectful families in order to be safe (American Academy of Pediatrics, 1996; Bassuk & Rubin, 1987; Kurtz, Hick-Coolick, Jarvis, & Kurtz, 1996). It is not feasible for many of the youths to return home due to poor relationships with their family of origin. While youths under the age of 18 may become wards of the state, making them eligible for services, many remain non-wards and are forced to fend for themselves on the streets, placing them at risk for assault or other unsafe situations. They develop identities and habits that assist them in negotiating and surviving the culture on the streets or in shelters. These adolescents have limited opportunities to develop life skills that promote mainstream roles such as that of student, family member or worker.

Domestic Violence

Domestic violence affects nearly five million women annually in the United States (U.S. Department of Justice), impacting them both medically and functionally. Victims of domestic violence are typically provided with shelter, financial and legal services, while important life skills are not addressed (C. Helfrich & Aviles, 2002). Women report substantial difficulty with daily activities (Gorde, Helfrich, & Finlayson, 2004). These women often lack life skills because they have not had the opportunity to acquire these skills or because the abuser typically controlled the household, allowing the woman little opportunity for responsibility and decision-making. Women may also lack confidence to access existing skills that would help establish independence. Autonomy is unfamiliar territory for survivors of domestic violence and therefore may be perceived as potentially unpredictable, uncomfortable or unsafe. These women are an underserved population, often not eligible for many rehabilitation programs where life skills might be taught. Further, the literature documents that women may be unable to access services that are available because of barriers such as lack of transportation, service provider's inadequate resources, or cost (Gallop & Everett, 2001; McCauley et al., 1995).

Mental Illness

Of the 3.5 million people in the U.S. who experience homelessness each year (The Urban Institute, 2000), 61-91% have psychiatric disabilities. These people spend more days homeless, rate their quality of life lower than those without mental illness, and have marked problems meeting basic needs (Sullivan, Burnam, Koegel, & Hollenberg, 2000). Mental health consumers and their families report a need for improved independent living skills (Hatfield, Fiersten, & Johnson, 1982; Solomon & Marcenko, 1992). Consumers lose housing after not paying rent because of inadequate finances, cognitive or behavioral limitations, difficulty managing on a low budget, the inability to successfully complete instrumental activities of daily living, isolation, lack of meaningful occupations or inadequate preparation (Cairns, 2001). The relationship of psychiatric symptoms to functional impairment is often overlooked even though symptoms affect individuals' personal health and lives, as well as their functioning and productivity in personal and vocational areas (Goodman, Saxe, & Harvey, 1991; Gorde, Helfrich, & Finlayson, 2004; Sullivan, Burnam, Koegel, & Hollenberg, 2000).

Mental illness has a profound and significant impact on an individual's ability to become and remain independent. The effects of mental illness are varied and often impair one's ability to engage in social interactions (Carlson, McNutt, Choi, & Rose, 2002), perform activities of daily living (Calysn, Morse, Klinkenberg, Yonker, & Trusty, 2002; Constantino, Sekula, Rabin, & Stone, 2000; Gilson, DePoy, & Cramer, 2001; Nedd, 2001; Schutt & Goldfinger, 1996) and manage individual and community responsibilities (Lindhorst, 2001; Riger & Krieglstein, 2000) in a manner that allows for both basic and instrumental needs to be met. Among the homeless population, the effects of mental illness are compounded by the difficulties that result from a lack of stable, safe and supportive housing and employment opportunities. This often results in an increased reliance on public assistance and an inability to attain economic independence (Lloyd & Taluc, 1999; Riger, Raja, & Camacho, 2002). Cognitive impairments are most common in individuals with schizophrenia and are found to be more severe than in other mental disorders and remain a stable aspect of the disorder, thus requiring accommodation rather than rehabilitation (Silverstein, Schenkel, Valone, & Nuernberger, 1998).

Study Purpose

The purpose of this study was to develop, implement and evaluate a life skills intervention with homeless individuals to optimize their housing independence by increasing their knowledge and use of life skills. A secondary purpose was to understand the demographic profiles of these three groups of homeless individuals and the pragmatics of conducting this type of research in order to make recommendations for more effective interventions.

METHODS

Need for Study

In several studies noted below, the authors conducted participatory needs assessments by asking individuals living in homeless shelters what they saw as their own needs. The youths perceived themselves lacking the most basic skills relevant to establishing stability in their lives. They reported not knowing how to manage money, locate safe and permanent housing, or to properly seek employment (Aviles, 2001). As noted earlier, women who experienced domestic violence had difficulty managing their finances, working towards their goals, finding a place to live and take care of themselves, identifying a place where they could be productive, and obtaining basic supplies (C. Helfrich & Gorde, 2002). Persons with mental illness identified not knowing how to manage money, food and nutrition, and room and self-care. The staff working with each group identified similar needs. Given this data, the following skills were selected for this set of interventions: employment (youth), financial management (female DV survivors) and food and nutrition (mentally ill adults). These skills are important to acquire while in the shelter in order to be independent afterwards (Roth, 2000). Because of the focus on emergency needs in the shelter, the participants have few opportunities to learn these important life skills.

Study Design

This project implemented and evaluated a life skills intervention for homeless individuals using a group pretest-posttest design. Study participants completed an initial life skills evaluation and then participated in four weekly group and individual sessions with an occupational therapist.

At the completion of the four-week module, a posttest was administered to assess knowledge attainment. Data were analyzed using descriptive statistics.

Services provided to homeless individuals must be based on empowerment theory rather than a traditional rehabilitation service model. Rehabilitation services are often dominated by an expert model (Feinstein, 1973) that subtly coerces clients, and results in a "collision of principles" between providers and clients (Trostle, 1988). In contrast, empowerment theory stresses self-reliance and reliance on peer networks in solving problems (Rappaport, 1994). Responsive services must be individually designed, culturally relevant, and respectful of the strengths, concerns, and needs of clients. Being client-centered means that services are based on consumer choices and preferences rather than only on provider judgments (Bond, 1998). The life skills intervention was designed so that individualized components could be implemented to maximize each client's strengths, address perceived obstacles, facilitate successful experiences, and allow for the forward movement and regression that often accompany change (Bandura, 1986; Prochaska, Norcross, & DiClemente, 1994; Regenold, Sherman, & Fenzel, 1999). The intervention incorporated an empowerment approach that encourages clients to be active and engaged in the creation and delivery of their own services (F. Balcazar, Keys, & Garate-Serafini, 1995; F. E. Balcazar, Keys, Kaplan, & Suarez-Balcazar, 1998; F. E. Balcazar, Keys, & Suarez-Balcazar, 2001).

Previous work with these populations allowed us to understand that service availability does not equate to service utilization (Gorde, Helfrich, & Finlayson, 2004). We surveyed participants to identify key factors that would facilitate use of services (Aviles, 2001). First, they felt that some services available to them were not relevant or valuable and wanted programs to address their stated needs and priorities. Second, they indicated that given the other demands on their time, any service should occur in a concentrated block once a week. Finally, parents with children identified the need for child care if they were to attend a program. To address these issues we: (a) designed a program that reflected their priorities and stated needs and that could be individually tailored to each individual, (b) offered the program in an appropriate format once a week, and (c) provided child care for those who were parents.

Settings

Each subpopulation of study participants came from a different shelter in a large Midwestern city. Youths were recruited from a citywide shelter that serves non-ward youth aged 14-21, primarily from economically disadvantaged families and neighborhoods. The facility provides a safe place for youths to stay while they find a permanent home and become economically self-sufficient. There are 16 beds and five cribs. The length of stay ranges from 1-120 days. The youths are expected to be out of the shelter during the day looking for housing and jobs and obtaining the necessary identification papers and documents to access services.

Domestic violence survivors were recruited from two sites, a transitional housing program and an emergency shelter operated by the same agency. The two-year transitional housing program serves 22 women and children. Women are required to be in school, training or work. The emergency shelter houses 32 residents with a three-month maximum length of stay.

Adults with mental illness were residents of an emergency housing program operated by an academic medical center psychiatry department. The program provides supervised, structured and protected living for 23 homeless mentally ill adults experiencing an acute psychiatric episode. Staff are on-site 24 hours. The average length of stay is 3-4 months. All residents have a documented psychiatric disability and 56% have a co-occurring substance abuse diagnosis.

The site populations are primarily African Americans who have incomes below the federal poverty guidelines and receive Medicaid. Although programming includes basic supportive services, social services and transitional services, the life skills that are taught by shelter staff are broad in scope and presented in a general manner. Life skills are not taught in a way that allows individual training, repetitive practice and ongoing coaching that is needed for persons who have cognitive limitations to acquire skills sufficient for independent living.

Participants

Participants were recruited from each site with the assistance of shelter staff. Flyers were posted in public areas of each setting and the interventionist attended weekly meetings to explain the project, answer questions and recruit potential participants. In order to provide individuals with autonomy, case managers were not involved in the recruitment process. To participate, subjects had to self-identify a life skill need, be willing to engage in a 60-minute group and a 60-minute individual session each week and be able to give informed consent. Additionally, all adults with mental illness were screened to verify their competence to give informed consent using the MacArthur Competence Assessment Tool for Clinical Research (Appelbaum, 2001). The only exclusion criteria were inability to understand English or participate in a 60-minute group. Participants, except for the adults with mental illnesses, who completed the entire four-week module were given a $10 grocery store gift certificate. The difference in reimbursement among the groups was due to the projects being funded by different grants. The University of Illinois Institutional Review Board and the Boards of each study site approved all aspects of the study.

For the adolescents and adults with mental illness, the life skills sessions were an add-on to the existing program. In the domestic violence shelter, participation in the intervention assisted some residents in meeting the required number of group and individual contact hours as determined by the shelter. All participants attending the sessions were voluntary and individuals could discontinue participation at any time without consequence to the services they would receive at the agency. The facilitators of the life skills intervention were third-year students in entry-level masters, or a post-professional master program in occupational therapy. All facilitators received supervision from one of the licensed authors.

Project Implementation

Following informed consent, the participants met individually with the occupational therapy interventionist who conducted an initial assessment for the intervention and developed goals with each participant. The Ansell-Casey Life Skills Assessment (ACLSA), a self-report tool, was administered to all interested individuals to determine life skill need, intervention eligibility and a baseline measure (Ansell & Casey Family Programs, 2005). The ACLSA assesses daily living skills (food and nutrition management), housing and community resources, money management, self-care, social development and work skills. The tool has four age-specific versions that represent development of life skills. The ACLSA generates three data scores: Mastery scores measure general life skill development, Performance scores measure ability to select accurate information and Benchmark scores compare individual performance to others of similar ages. The ACLSA demonstrates acceptable internal consistency reliability, content validity, construct validity and test-retest reliability (Nollan, Horn, Downs, & Pecora, 2000, 2002). The ACLSA subscales were readministered at the end of the intervention module to measure changes in knowledge and skill performance.

Program Description

The intervention was based on the Model of Human Occupation (Kielhofner, 2002) and consisted of eight 60-minute contacts: four provided in a group format and four individual sessions. The intervention lasted four weeks with a group and individual session scheduled each week. The individual sessions were designed to supplement the content provided in the groups and were scheduled at the convenience of the participants.

At the start of each weekly group session, participants were provided with activity packets containing resource materials for the group. The physical environment was arranged to include both participants and facilitator as equally integral parts of the group. For example, chairs were placed in a circle to encourage discussion. This was ultimately intended to promote a collaborative group atmosphere and social learning. The occupational therapy interventionist facilitated the activities and discussion for the designated week's topic and encouraged participants to direct the discussion topics whenever possible. The interventionist provided redirection only as necessary in order to maintain group norms and cover the weekly topics.

After each group, participants completed a quiz to evaluate content retention and select individual session topics. Quiz answers were discussed with each participant during individual sessions. Since these sessions addressed the needs and interests of each participant, topics and activities varied greatly. In general, the content of individual sessions was determined by the participants and provided a means for further exploration and hands-on practice of large group topics. For example, one participant identified a need to learn how to read food labels and make healthier food choices while another participant wanted to learn how to make microwave pasta.

Tables 1-3 provide a listing of the session topics covered in each module. All participants engaged in the same group discussion topics and activities. Individual sessions addressed individual needs identified from a predetermined list of goals each participant prioritized at the end of the group session quiz. Participants could set a related goal that was not on the list.

TABLE 1. Finding Employment–Youth Intervention

Week	Group Sessions	Individual Sessions
1	**Introduction to Employment** Identifying career interests Understanding the importance of employment Workplace technology	Chores & responsibilities prep for a job How interests & skills match career choices Current job interests/gaining experience Making realistic vocational/work goals Aspects you like about your job
2	**Learning How to Search for Employment** Finding a part-time job in the community Performing a search for employment	Reading ads for jobs in the newspaper Recognizing different ways to look for a job Practicing using the internet to locate a job Practicing completing a job application Documents required in applying for a job
3	**Skills Required for a Job** Cover letter & resume Interviewing skills Job interview follow up	Practicing a mock interview Creating a resume Writing a cover letter Learning about interviewing
4	**Job Maintenance & Advancement** Employee wage deductions, benefits, rights Characteristics of a good employee Knowing how & why to change jobs	Handling situations when in charge Using office equipment Wages & prevailing wage act Job safety & health protections rights Getting along with the boss Changing jobs Good workplace attitude Advancing in the workplace Reading a pay-check stub

RESULTS

Demographics

Seventy-three residents enrolled in the life skills interventions. The three sites reflect that the majority of the participants, 86.3% (63) were female with 72% youth, 100% abused women and 61.5% adults with mental illness being female. The ages of the residents range from 17-55 years; mean ages of each group were youth (19 years), abused women (31.28 years) and the adults with mental illness (45.77 years). Ethnicity was:

TABLE 2. Managing Your Finances–Domestic Violence Victims Intervention

Week	Group Sessions	Individual Sessions
1	**Introduction to Financial Management** How values influence money decisions Making money last	Saving money Cutting down on expenses Developing a monthly budget Investing money How I spend my money each week How much money I need each week
2	**Money Management** Ways to shop on a budget Advertising's impact on spending	Purchasing items on sale Knowing unit pricing Making payments Strategies for grocery shopping
3	**Savings & Checking Accounts** Long term savings goal Services provided by financial institutions Electronic banking Cashing checks & borrowing money Opening & maintaining a savings/checking account	Maintaining a checking account Applying for a loan Getting a car loan Learning about savings accounts Writing checks Checking accounts Using an ATM Using money orders
4	**Projecting a Budget** Developing a realistic spending plan for a month Pros and cons of using credit Importance of developing and maintaining a sound credit hx & credit rating	Strategies to pay bills on time & consequences of not paying on time Saving receipts to help manage your budget Income & expenses related to budget Developing a personal budget Differences between credit cards Reading a pay stub

13.7% (10) Caucasian, 71.2% (52) Black, 6.8% (5) Hispanic, 5.5% (4) Biracial, 1.4% (1) Native American and 1.4% (1) other. The length of stay in each shelter varied with respect to duration (1-491 days) and mean number of days (102.3) sheltered. Psychiatric conditions were reported by 44.5% youth, 21% abused women and 100% of the adults with mental illness and physical conditions were reported by no youth, 19.1% (8) abused women and 69.2% (9) adults with mental illness.

Socioeconomically, 72% youth, 67% abused women and 92% adults with mental illness earned at least a high-school degree or graduate equivalent. The majority of the participants (72% youth, 79% abused women and 100% adults with mental illness) were unemployed; however, all par-

TABLE 3. Food and Nutrition–Adults with Mental Illness Intervention

Week	Group Sessions	Individual Sessions
1	**Introduction to food management** Eating on a limited budget Stretching the food dollar Comparing cost & nutrition of fast food & healthy alternatives	Setting personal meal budget Evaluating personal spending habits Improving ways to shop smart Improving assertiveness skills Touring a Soup Kitchen/Food Pantry *Learning to microwave cook
2	**Nutrition Basics** Understanding "Food Pyramid" Planning variety in diet Diet related illnesses & statistics My own eating habits Determining a staples list	How medication & health impact eating Developing realistic eating & nutritional goals Strategies to maintain a less harmful diet Recognizing personal eating habits *How to increase interest in food
3	**Food Safety & Kitchen Care** Buying/Preparing/Cooking/ Eating/Storing food safely Cleaning up Choose a meal to cook	Preparing a meal Reviewing specific food safety concerns Creating a kitchen chore list *Making microwave pasta Creating personal hygiene goals
4	**Meal Preparation** Planning a meal Preparing a meal Microwave & No cook meals Microwave cooking Portion sizing & leftovers Cleaning up	Planning for future needs Safety while cooking Identifying meal preparation goals *Making microwave pasta Understanding how to read recipe

*Goal identified by participant

ticipants noted some previous work experience. Source of income varied among the subgroups; women with children were eligible for more resources.

Intervention Results

Due to the transience of this population, 32 of the 73 participants completed pre- and posttests including six youths, 13 women who experienced domestic violence and 13 adults with mental illness. The pretest scores of the 41 individuals who did not complete the entire study were compared to those who did, and no significant differences were found. Descriptively, the group demonstrated an increase in mastery scores over time. Twenty (62%) module completers had an increase in their mastery scores, 16% (5) demonstrated no change and 22% (7) demonstrated a decrease in scores. Despite the descriptive changes, there were no statistically significant changes in the groups of youth or adults with mental illness. However, despite the small sample size of women who experienced domestic violence, paired t-tests demonstrated statistically significant changes ($t = -3.898$, $df = 12$, $p = .002$).

DISCUSSION

Demographically the study sample was more diverse than expected. Participants had life experiences prior to becoming homeless that included a range of educational and employment backgrounds. Health issues in homeless populations may be undetected due to lack of access to health care; however, the youth may not have yet developed medical issues and the adults with mental illness were living in a shelter operated by a medical center where a physical examination was required and made available at a medical clinic housed in the same building as the shelter. This diversity of life experiences highlights the complexities of the homeless population. They do not fit the stereotype that many people expect them to. For a variety of reasons, many quite complicated, the study participants have found themselves living in a shelter with very little resources to draw from.

The Ansell-Casey Life Skill Assessment and Quiz scores indicate that participants were impacted by the intervention. Lower scores on the posttest may not necessarily indicate a decline in ability. Instead, they may indicate an increased accuracy in one's self-appraisal of skills from learning what one does and does not know. A limitation of this study is the population transience, which affected the high drop-out rate and power of the quantitative analyses. A detailed discussion of the scorès and their meaning has been reported elsewhere (C. A. Helfrich, Aviles, Badiani, Walens, & Sabol, under review). Clinically, the ACLSA scores were useful for providing feedback to participants before the intervention; however, pre- and posttests specific to the content of each module would have been more useful and informative. While the quantitative data outcomes of this study were limited due to the sample size, the qualitative findings were informative and have applicability to other programs.

The remainder of this section discusses the challenges that were encountered by the researchers, interventionists and onsite staff and the strategies that were developed to overcome those challenges. Strategies were developed to address challenges and were categorized by their target focus: staff, participants or the environment. Each category with recommendations for implementation is discussed below.

Staff

At each site we identified key staff and developed relationships with them so we became partners in the intervention and research process, rather than one party being an obstacle to the other. Both onsite staff members and researchers had the potential to get in each other's way or interfere with ongoing processes. To facilitate the partnership we educated staff about the project and relevant aspects of the research; for example, IRB imposed limitations on communication. We also tried to understand the nuances of the site to better appreciate the impact our presence had on the staff. These tasks were accomplished through regular individual meetings with key staff as well as through presentation to the larger staff group.

Recommendations

1. Remember that research and clinical practice is a balancing act: Clarity of information sharing is critical. Discuss what research and clinical information can be shared, with whom, and at what points it can be shared.
2. Develop processes for sharing urgent or critical information: Remember the bottom line is ALWAYS client safety.
3. Maintain a healthy respect for onsite staff expertise: Staff who work with the population every day have knowledge and insight, an offsite clinician does not.

Participants

Recruiting participants and maintaining them throughout the study was limited by characteristics and transience of the three populations. The onsite interventionist attended client meetings (house meetings, community meetings, groups) to advertise the project to potential participants. She was also available afterwards to answer questions. This approach was useful because it allowed for face-to-face contact and provided an opportunity to address questions and concerns; however, it was not enough. Informal interactions with clients in the day room or in the halls provided additional opportunities to build rapport. That rapport helped the interventionist to meet clients where they were at when they entered the study. Once a client was in the study, she also took opportunities to provide additional information during individual sessions on topics of interest such as employment possibilities or free recreational information. Finally, because these pilot studies were grant-funded, we were able to offer a small financial incentive to participants at two of the sites which increased the attractiveness of the intervention.

Recommendations

1. Select interventionist from onsite staff if possible.
2. Encourage word-of-mouth referrals: Past participants are better marketers of the intervention than clinical experts.
3. Present the least amount of information necessary to teach a skill: Everyone reaches a saturation point and people under stress reach that point sooner.
4. Acknowledge completion of the intervention through Certificates of Completion: This may be the individual's first "completed" activity.

Environment

Environmental challenges required flexibility and creativity to overcome the space and time limitations encountered by the interventionist. The interventionists, who were all full-time students, were able to be flexible with their schedules in order to accommodate the client's requests to have group on a particular day or time. Because each program had their own set of scheduled requirements, many participants had busy schedules which often conflicted with the group schedule. The interventionist was flexible with the frequency of scheduled groups (once or twice per week) and the length of individual sessions (1-2 hours) to meet the needs of particular groups of participants. Flexibility was also required if someone missed a group session. In these cases individual sessions were scheduled to make up the material.

Recommendations

1. Use preestablished group times: Reinforce established habits and routines.
2. Be consistent with interventionist, place and time of group.
3. Maintain the group experience as much as possible: Missed group content can be conveyed in an individual session, but the group process cannot.

CONCLUSION

This study demonstrated the complexity of the homeless population and usefulness of occupational therapy interventions to improve the life skills of homeless persons. The study elucidated a number of challenges encountered by researchers and clinicians who collaborated to provide a clinical outcomes study in shelter settings. Strategies developed by the research team in collaboration with the clinical sites allowed the intervention to be delivered effectively and provided useful information for future studies. More research is needed to fully understand the most effective methods and interventions for improving the life skills of homeless individuals. Occupational therapists are encouraged to collaborate with shelters to provide needed life skill interventions.

REFERENCES

American Academy of Pediatrics (1996). Health needs of homeless children and families. *Pediatrics*, 98(4), 789-791.

Ansell, D. I., & Casey Family Programs. (2005). *The Ansell Casey Life Skills Assessment IV*. Seattle, WA: Dorothy I. Ansell and Casey Family Programs.

Appelbaum, P. S., & Grisso, T. (2001). *MacArthur Competence Assessment Tool for Clinical Research*. Sarasota: Professional Resource Press.

Aviles, A. (2001). *Service needs: Insights from homeless youth*. Unpublished Master's thesis, University of Illinois at Chicago, Department of Occupational Therapy, Chicago.

Balcazar, F., Keys, C., & Garate-Serafini, J. (1995). Learning to recruit assistance to attain transition goals: A program for adjudicated youths with disabilities. *Remedial and Special Education*, 16, 237-246.

Balcazar, F. E., Keys, C. B., Kaplan, D. L., & Suarez-Balcazar, Y. (1998). Participatory action research and people with disabilities: Principles and challenges. *Canadian Journal of Rehabilitation*, 12, 105-112.

Balcazar, F. E., Keys, C. B., & Suarez-Balcazar, Y. (2001). Empowering Latinos with disabilities to address issues of independent living and disability rights: A capacity building approach. *Journal of Prevention & Intervention in the Community*, 21(2), 53-70.

Bandura, A. (1986). *Social foundations of thought and action: A social cognitive theory*. Englewood Cliffs, NJ: Prentice Hall.

Bassuk, E. L., & Rubin, L. (1987). Homeless children: A neglected population. *American Journal of Orthopsychiatry*, 57, 278-287.

Bond, G. R. (1998). Principles of the individual placement and support model: Empirical support. *Psychiatric Rehabilitation Journal*, 22(1), 11-23.

Cairns, P. (2001). Life skills training for homeless people: A review of the evidence. *Precis: A summary series of recent research commissioned by Scottish Homes*, 141.

Calysn, R. J., Morse, G. A., Klinkenberg, W. D., Yonker, R. D., & Trusty, M. L. (2002). Moderators and mediators of client satisfaction in case management programs for clients with severe mental illness. *Mental Health Services Research*, 4(4), 267-275.

Carlson, B. E., McNutt, L., Choi, D. Y., & Rose, I. M. (2002). Intimate partner abuse and mental health: The role of social support and other protective factors. *Violence Against Women*, 8, 720-745.

Constantino, R. E., Sekula, L. E., Rabin, B., & Stone, C. (2000). Negative life experiences, depression, and immune function in abused and non-abused women. *Biological Research for Nursing*, 1, 190-198.

Davis, L. V., Hagen, J. L., & Early, T. J. (1994). Social services for battered women: Are they adequate, accessible, and appropriate? *Social Work*, 39(6), 695-704.

Ensign, J. G. J. (1998). Health and access to care: Perspectives of homeless youth in Baltimore City, U.S.A. *Social Science & Medicine*, 47(12), 2087-2099.

Feinstein, A. (1973). An analysis of diagnostic reasoning, Parts I and II. *Yale Journal of Biology and Medicine*, 46, 212-232, 264-283.

First, R. J., Rife, J. C., & Kraus, S. (1990). Case management with people who are homeless and mentally ill: Preliminary findings from an NIMH demonstration project. *Psychosocial Rehabilitation Journal*, 14(2), 87-91.

Folsom, D., & Jeste, D. V. (2002). Schizophrenia in homeless persons: A systematic review of the literature. *Acta Psychiatrica Scandinavica*, 105(6), 404-413.

Gallop, R., & Everett, B. (2001). Recognizing the signs and symptoms. In B. Everett & R. Gallop (Eds.), *The link between childhood trauma & mental illness: Effective interventions for mental health professionals* (pp. 57-79). Thousand Oaks, CA: Sage Publications.

Gilson, S. F., DePoy, E., & Cramer, E. P. (2001). Linking the assessment of self-reported functional capacity with abuse experiences of women with disabilities. *Violence Against Women*, 7(4), 418-431.

Goodman, L., Saxe, L., & Harvey, M. (1991). Homelessness as psychological trauma: Broadening perspectives. *American Psychologist*, 46(11), 1219-1225.

Gorde, M., Helfrich, C. A., & Finlayson, M. L. (2004). Trauma symptoms and life skill needs of domestic violence victims. *Journal of Interpersonal Violence*, 19(6), 691-708.

Gutmann, D. (1975). Parenthood: A key to comparative study of life cycle. In N. Datan & L. E. Ginsberg (Eds.), *Lifespan development psychology*. New York: Academic Press.

Hatfield, A. B., Fiersten, R., & Johnson, D. M. (1982). Meeting the needs of families of the psychiatrically disabled. *Psychosocial Rehabilitation Journal*, 6(1), 27-40.

Helfrich, C., & Aviles, A. (2002). *Longitudinal service use of domestic violence survivors: A two-year study*. Paper presented at the MCDV 2002: First National Conference on Medical Care and Domestic Violence, Dallas, TX.

Helfrich, C., & Gorde, M. (2002). *Trauma symptoms and life skill needs across domestic violence service delivery settings*. Paper presented at the MCDV 2002: First National Conference on Medical Care and Domestic Violence, Dallas, TX.

Helfrich, C. A. (2001). *Domestic abuse across the lifespan: The role of occupational therapy*. West Hazelton, PA: The Haworth Press, Inc.

Helfrich, C. A., Aviles, A. M., Badiani, C., Walens, D., & Sabol, P. (under review). Life skills interventions with homeless people: Outcomes and strategies.

Kannenberg, K., & Boyer, D. (1997). Occupational therapy update. Occupational therapy evaluation and intervention in an employment program for homeless youths. *Psychiatric Services*, 48, 631-633.

Kielhofner, G. (2002). *A model of human occupation: Theory and application* (3rd ed). Baltimore: Lippincott Williams and Wilkins.

Kurtz, P., Hick-Coolick, A., Jarvis, S., & Kurtz, G. (1996). Assessment of abuse in runaway and homeless youth. *Child and Youth Care Forum*, 25(3), 183-194.

Lindhorst, T. P. (2001). The effect of domestic violence on welfare use, employment and mental health: A quantitative and qualitative analysis. *Dissertation Abstracts International*, 62(6-A), 2239.

Lloyd, S., & Taluc, N. (1999). The effects of male violence on female employment. *Violence Against Women*. 5(370-392).

McCauley, J., Kern, D., Kolodner, K., Dill, L., Schroeder, A., De Chant, H. et al. (1995). The "battering syndrome": Prevalence and clinical characteristics of domestic violence in primary care internal medicine practices. *Annals of Internal Medicine*, 123(10), 737-746.

National Coalition for the Homeless. Retrieved February 22, 2005, from http://www.nationalhomeless.org

Nedd, D. M. (2001). Self-reported health status and depression of battered black women. *The Association of Black Nursing Faculty Journal*, 12, 32-35.

Nollan, K. A., Horn, M., Downs, A. C., & Pecora, P. J. (2000, 2002). *Ansell-Casey Life Skills Assessment (ACLSA) and Life Skills Guidebook Manual*. Seattle, WA: Casey Family Programs.

Prochaska, J., Norcross, J., & DiClemente, C. (1994). *Changing for good: The revolutionary program that explains the six stages of change and teaches you how to free yourself from bad habits.* New York: W. Morrow.

Rappaport, J. (1994). Empowerment as a guide to doing research: Diversity as a positive value. In E. J. Trickett, R. J. Watts, & E. Birman (Eds.), *Human diversity: Perspectives on people in context* (pp. 404-423). San Francisco, CA: Jossey-Bass Inc.

Regenold, M., Sherman, M. F., & Fenzel, M. (1999). Getting back to work: Self-efficacy as a predictor of employment outcome. *Psychiatric Rehabilitation Journal*, 22(4), 361-367.

Riger, S., & Krieglstein, M. (2000). The impact of welfare reform on men's violence against women. *American Journal of Community Psychology*, 28(5), 631-647.

Riger, S., Raja, S., & Camacho, J. (2002). The radiating impact of intimate partner violence. *Journal of Interpersonal Violence*, 17(2), 184-205.

Roth, J., & Brooks-Gunn, J. (2000). What do adolescents need for healthy development? Implications for youth policy. *Social Policy Report, Giving Child and Youth Development Knowledge Away*, 14(1), 3-19.

Schutt, R. K., & Goldfinger, S. M. (1996). Housing preferences and perceptions of health and functioning among homeless mentally ill persons. *Psychiatric Services*, 47(4), 381-386.

Shordike, A., & Howell, D. (2001). The reindeer of hope: An occupational therapy program in a homeless shelter. *Occupational Therapy in Health Care*, 15, 57-68.

Silverstein, S. M., Schenkel, L. S., Valone, C., & Nuernberger, S. W. (1998). Cognitive deficits and psychiatric rehabilitation outcomes in schizophrenia. *Psychiatric Quarterly*, 69(3), 169-191.

Solomon, P., & Marcenko, M. (1992). Families of adults with severe mental illness: Their satisfaction with inpatient and outpatient treatment. *Psychosocial Rehabilitation Journal*, 16(1), 121-132.

Substance Abuse and Mental Health Services Administration (2003). *Blueprint for change: Ending chronic homelessness for persons with serious mental illness and/ or co-occurring substance abuse disorders.* Rockville, MD: U.S. Department of Health & Human Services.

Sullivan, G., Burnam, A., Koegel, P., & Hollenberg, J. (2000). Quality of life of homeless persons with mental illness: Results from the course-of-homelessness study. *Psychiatric Services*, 51(9), 1135-1141.

The Urban Institute (2000). *A new look at homelessness in America.*

Trostle, J. A. (1988). Medical complicance as an ideology. *Social Science and Medicine*, 27(12), 1299-1308.

Tryssenaar, J., Jones, E. J., & Lee, D. (1999). Occupational performance needs of a shelter population. *Canadian Journal of Occupational Therapy*, 66(4), 188-196.

U.S. Department of Justice. Extent, nature and consequences of intimate partner violence. Retrieved September 6, 2001, from http://www.ojp.usdoj.gov/nij.html

doi:10.1300/J003v20n03_12

Index

Page numbers followed by "t" denote tables.

© 2006 by The Haworth Press, Inc. All rights reserved.

BOOK ORDER FORM!

Order a copy of this book with this form or online at:
http://www.HaworthPress.com/store/product.asp?sku= 5960

Homelessness in America

Perspectives, Characterizations, and Considerations for Occupational Therapy

___ in softbound at $26.00 ISBN-13: 978-0-7890-3192-1 / ISBN-10: 0-7890-3192-2.
___ in hardbound at $42.00 ISBN-13: 978-0-7890-3191-4 / ISBN-10: 0-7890-3191-4.

COST OF BOOKS ________

POSTAGE & HANDLING ________
US: $4.00 for first book & $1.50 for each additional book
Outside US: $5.00 for first book & $2.00 for each additional book.

SUBTOTAL ________

In Canada: add 6% GST. ________

STATE TAX ________
CA, IL, IN, MN, NJ, NY, OH, PA & SD residents please add appropriate local sales tax.

FINAL TOTAL ________
If paying in Canadian funds, convert using the current exchange rate, UNESCO coupons welcome.

❑ **BILL ME LATER:**
Bill-me option is good on US/Canada/Mexico orders only; not good to jobbers, wholesalers, or subscription agencies.

❑ **Signature** ________

❑ **Payment Enclosed: $**________

❑ **PLEASE CHARGE TO MY CREDIT CARD:**

❑ Visa ❑ MasterCard ❑ AmEx ❑ Discover
❑ Diner's Club ❑ Eurocard ❑ JCB

Account #________

Exp Date________

Signature________
(Prices in US dollars and subject to change without notice.)

PLEASE PRINT ALL INFORMATION OR ATTACH YOUR BUSINESS CARD

Name ________

Address ________

City ________ State/Province ________ Zip/Postal Code ________

Country ________

Tel ________ Fax ________

E-Mail ________

May we use your e-mail address for confirmations and other types of information? ❑Yes ❑No We appreciate receiving your e-mail address. Haworth would like to e-mail special discount offers to you, as a preferred customer. **We will never share, rent, or exchange your e-mail address.** We regard such actions as an invasion of your privacy.

Order from your **local bookstore** or directly from
The Haworth Press, Inc. 10 Alice Street, Binghamton, New York 13904-1580 • USA
Call our toll-free number (1-800-429-6784) / Outside US/Canada: (607) 722-5857
Fax: 1-800-895-0582 / Outside US/Canada: (607) 771-0012
E-mail your order to us: orders@HaworthPress.com

For orders outside US and Canada, you may wish to order through your local sales representative, distributor, or bookseller.
For information, see http://HaworthPress.com/distributors

(Discounts are available for individual orders in US and Canada only, not booksellers/distributors.)

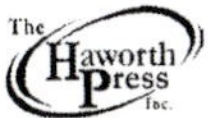

Please photocopy this form for your personal use.
www.HaworthPress.com

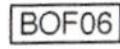